What other health care professionals are saying about the DMR Method®

"I'm a neurosurgeon who specializes in complicated brain and spine surgery. Although I am a surgeon my first course of action with every patient is to consider all non-surgical treatments when appropriate. For many spinal conditions I've found that the DMR Method produces consistent results and has an amazing ability to help patients avoid surgery. Even when a patient has previously had spinal surgery, the DMR Method can be valuable in helping that person stabilize their spine and prevent a recurrence of symptoms and additional surgery. I also appreciate how they've built specific procedures into the DMR Method to help identify when a surgery consult might be helpful. Their team approach, with chiropractors and physical therapists working with other medical specialists to get a person well, is commendable. When I've worked with patients they've referred to me, I'm always impressed with how educated and motivated they are. This book will strengthen a patient's knowledge and help them understand their condition, the best treatment options, what they can do on their own, how to avoid surgery, and when it's time to consider surgery. It's a testament to the effectiveness of the DMR Method that most patients I refer for treatment do not need to return for surgery. This book is the next step in the development of the innovative DMR Method."

- John C. Mullan, MD

"As a practicing orthopaedic surgeon for over 20 years, I am always looking for ways to improve and expedite my patients' recovery. Whenever possible, conservative treatment options are explored to hopefully prevent the need for surgery. Over the last several years I have worked with the chiropractors and physical therapists that developed the DMR method. I have found this to be a well-conceived and structured systematic approach to the evaluation and treatment of many conditions and especially useful in the treatment of several spine disorders. The greatest benefit of the DMR method is that patients receive a personalized treatment program that is designed specifically for them and for their problem. They are thoroughly involved in the treatment plan and receive supervised care. The DMR Method book is an excellent resource for patients to help guide them through nonoperative management of their specific issue and also discusses when surgery should be considered for their condition. Many patients have benefited from the DMR approach and method and have found this to be an extremely valuable program."

- Douglas A. Becker, MD

"Dr. Pete L'Allier first introduced me to the DMR method 8 years ago. I was impressed with this progressive unique spine treatment program which utilized the combined talents of chiropractors and physical therapists. Since then, we have collaborated on many clinical case studies using MRI to evaluate pre and post DMR treatment results. I continue to be enthusiastically impressed with the successful clinical outcomes experienced by patients participating in his programs.

Congratulations on your hard work, perseverance and teamwork in creating the DMR method."

- William J. Mullin, MD
Spine Radiologist

"As an internal medicine physician with substantial back pain from a herniated lumbar disc, I can attest to the effectiveness of the DMR approach. I believe strongly in nonsurgical approaches to back pain so naturally tried standard physical therapy alone without success for over half a year. The pain originating in my back and shooting down my leg had become unrelenting so a colleague suggested I try the DMR program. After completing this program I have required only minimal, periodic adjustment to remain pain free and have regained my active lifestyle. I would encourage anyone experiencing back pain to complete the DMR program."

- Andrew Maresh, DO

"I work with many patients who have serious spinal issues. Many times I work as a link between non-surgical care providers and surgeons. I always try to do everything possible to keep patients on the non-surgical side of care, which can be tricky sometimes because the spine is very complex. To add to the complexity, lifestyle factors often have a dramatic impact on the health of the spine and how that affects the ability of the patient to recover. For example, a person who smokes, drives a freight truck for a living, and spends their weekends up north working on their cabin has a completely different recovery potential than a person who works at a desk, goes to the health club three to four times per week, and spends their weekends running their kids to various sports activities. That's what I love about the DMR Method; in addition to identifying the root cause of a patient's condition and providing a well researched intelligent treatment plan, it also identifies and addresses the lifestyle factors that could have an impact on short-term and long-term recovery. The DMR Method book has all the self-care, lifestyle, and wellness resources organized in a user-friendly way that will make it easy for a patient to learn what to do and how to do it on their own. What a great resource for patients!"

- Dr. David Williams, DO
Internal Medicine / Critical Care

The DMR METHOD
Advanced Nonsurgical Care for Neck and Back Pain

Peter Wesley Thomas L'Allier

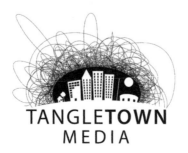

TANGLE**TOWN**
MEDIA

Disclaimer

The information in this book is intended for educational use only and should not be construed as medical advice. You should consult with your physician before attempting any activity or making any lifestyle changes discussed in this book. Although every attempt is made to ensure the accuracy of the information presented, the author and publisher are not liable for any illness or injury that may result from attempting any activities or lifestyle changes presented in this book.

The paper used in this publication meets the minimum requirements of the American National Standards for Information Services - Permanence of Paper for Printed Library Materials, ANSI Z39.48-1984.

Library of Congress Cataloging-in-Publication Data

L'Allier, Peter Wesley Thomas.
 The DMR method : non-surgical solution to severe back pain / Peter Wesley Thomas L'Allier.
     pages cm
 Includes bibliographical references and index.
 ISBN 978-1-933889-40-5 (alk. paper)
 1. Backache--Alternative treatment. 2. Neck pain--Alternative treatment. I. Title.
 RD771.B217L35 2015
 617.5'64--dc23
                          2014041530

Dedication

This book is dedicated to an amazing team of healthcare providers who collectively made this book possible. Over the last eight years, our collaboration, founded on mutual respect, trust, and a burning passion to help people get well, has resulted in a groundbreaking new system of evaluation and treatment for complicated spinal conditions. I have truly been blessed to work with such a professional, diverse, and good-hearted group of caregivers. My name may be on the cover of this book, but what you are about to read is the culmination of the knowledge and skill of literally dozens of caring, compassionate healthcare experts.

Acknowledgments

Numerous people were instrumental in developing the DMR Method. In addition to all the patients who participated in clinical case studies, I would like to acknowledge the following people and organizations for their expertise, knowledge, encouragement and support.:

Jim McDonald
John T. Beecher, MD, ABFP
Brownie E. Williams, D.C.
Lynne Hvidsten, DC
Ensor E. Transfeldt, MD
Barron Johnson, DC
Aimee Laurann Coulson
Jennifer Henke, DPT
Mehmet Oz, MD
David Leske, DC
Alex Fox, DC
Dan Kennedy
Brian Lund, DC
Stephanie E.Mussmann, DC, MS, DACBR
Jim Jennings
Douglas A. Becker, MD
Thomas J. Gilbert, Jr., M.D., M.P.P.
Timothy J. Mick, D.C., D.A.C.B.R., F.I.C.C
Mark Backlund
Amy Klausen Burge
Carrie Emery
John Moore
Kelly Kohler, MT
Stephanie Musselman
Kristin Wegner
Juliet Trow
Jeff Fitzloff
Michlynn Heide, DC

Tom Hutchinson
Loren Stoner, DC
Warren Moe, DC
Charles V. Burton, MD, F.A.C.S.
Frank David Harris LMT
Michelle Lelwica, DC
Jannel Kammerer, MPT
John Mullan, M.D.
Jeff Finn
Amanda Nelson, PTA
Greg Stanley
Laura Hoese, PA
Anna McConville, PT
Noelle Young, DPT
Zena Zander, DC
Rob Cherney
Robert H. Long, M.D.
William J. Mullin, M.D.
Kellie Stebe, DPT
Shannon Jones
Lisa Moy
Jerry Peterson
Peter Taunton
Phil Bolsta
Donna Woodall
Kelie Davis, DPT
Heather Ward, RT(R)
J.A. Schwartz, PT

Abby Bell, DC
Becca Cooper, LMT
Jose L'Allier, CPT
Brody Peterson, DC
Rachel Moore, DC
Nikki Vanecek, M.Ac.O.M., L.Ac.
Rebecca Hicks Photography
The Center for Diagnostic Imaging
Chattanooga Medical Supply, Inc
Todd Berntson, MA, DC, LPC

Trevor Northagen, DPT
Seth Perrier, CPT
Jaime Cupit, DPT
Shauna Alder, LMT
Chandani Amin, DPT
Paul Youngberg, PTA
Dynatronics
Neurosurgical Associates
Hopkins Snap Fitness

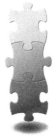

Table of Contents

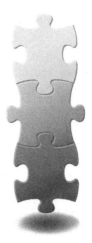

Introduction

Over the last twenty-five years, I've heard more than my share of stories from people struggling with back issues—the details of their injuries, what treatments they explored, their desperate search to find relief, how their struggles affected them and the people closest to them, and the often staggering costs they incurred. For many of them, no standard treatments—ranging from physical therapy to chiropractic to massage to medical pain management, and even to surgery—seemed to work. This puzzled me for many years because I knew that each of those treatments was scientifically valid and could be effective individually. I was determined to find the missing piece of the puzzle.

I spent years meeting with medical doctors, spine surgeons, physical therapists, and chiropractors about this problem. The message I consistently heard was that more communication and teamwork were needed between a patient's providers. Of course, the big question was how to achieve that. Four separate breakthroughs over the next three years produced the answer.

First, our team of knowledgeable and experienced physical therapists and chiropractors, with the help of some allied medical providers, developed the first standardized protocol of evaluation and treatment for the spine that combined physical therapy, chiropractic, and medical treatment. We reviewed research from all over the world, met with multiple spine care specialists and surgeons, and spent countless hours identifying key factors in nonsurgical treatment of complicated spinal conditions. We synthesized all that information to refine and continually improve this nonsurgical protocol, which we called the DMR (Diagnose, Manage and Rehabilitate) Method.

Our goals were to help people get out of pain, regain their physical abilities, prevent recurrence of the condition, and, most important, teach them how to effectively manage their condition on their own without resorting to surgery, injections, or other invasive procedures.

Second, a patient named Amy came into our clinic in 2007 with a severe disc herniation. Her debilitating lower back and right leg pain had been triggered when she bent over to pick up a laundry basket. Our clinical findings and the severity of her pain prompted me to recommend an MRI scan. The radiologist we referred her to at the Center for Diagnostic Imaging, one of the largest diagnostic imaging groups in the country, called us right after her MRI to tell us that Amy had a severe extruded disc herniation that required immediate surgical intervention. After examining the MRI scan myself and seeing how large the herniation was, I agreed with the radiologist and recommended to Amy that she see a surgeon as soon as possible.

The only person who didn't agree was Amy; she refused to even consider surgery. Given her resistance, I told her we could begin the DMR Method of treatment, but that if she didn't show rapid improvement she would have to get a surgical consult. Two weeks after starting the DMR Method, her leg pain was gone; by the eighth all of her symptoms were resolved.

When Amy's radiologist contacted me to see how her surgery had gone, I told him that she had opted to receive the DMR Method of treatment and that all of her symptoms had resolved. Surprised, he requested that we send her back for a follow-up MRI. That exam showed that the herniation had been completely reabsorbed.

Third, encouraged by Amy's recovery, the Center for Diagnostic Imaging offered to help us do a study utilizing pre- and post-MRI scans. We began with a pilot study that included twenty patients. Based on the outcomes of that study, we refined the DMR Method evaluation and treatment protocols and began the first DMR Method clinical case study. That study, completed in 2010, was one of the only clinical case studies of its kind in the country and was a rousing success. Fully 100 percent of the participants experienced a decrease in their symptoms; their functional abilities improved an average of 50 percent. Most important, 100 percent of the patients were able to avoid surgery. We now had proof that we were successfully treating cases that were previously thought to be treatable only by surgery.

That may sound astonishing, but it's important to understand that part of what makes the DMR Method so successful is that a portion of the protocol is an evaluation that helps us identify if a patient is a candidate for this integrative methodology. Unfortunately, some patients do need surgery, and it's our responsibility to diagnose those patients quickly and make appropriate

DMR Method™ Case Study

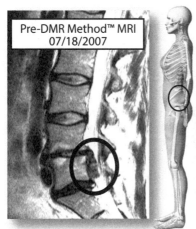

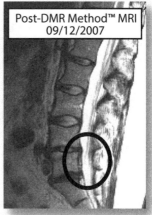

Severe Disc Herniation Lumbar Spine

Amy was loading her washing machine when she bent over to pick up a laundry basket. She felt something "go out" in her lower back and experienced an intense pain that began radiating down her left leg. Her leg pain soon progressed to numbness and weakness and she began to have difficulty walking. Based on MRI findings, medical radiologists recommended emergency surgery.

DIAGNOSIS

The MRI confirmed a severe extruded disc herniation at L4-5, causing nerve compression. DMR Method Evaluation revealed severe misalignment and immobility in the lower lumbar spine and pelvis, with severe muscle spasm and inflammation.

TREATMENT

Due to the severity of Amy's condition, her case was closely monitored. Her treatment following the completion of the Acute Lumbar DMR Protocol was focused on oscillating decompression traction, cold laser therapy and Integrated Progressive Mobilization (IPM).

OUTCOME

Amy experienced a resolution of all symptoms without needing surgery. Her extruded disc was entirely reabsorbed and she has been able to resume normal daily activities without pain. After seven years, Amy reports continued symptoms resolution and normal physical abilities.

NOTE: Amy was the very first DMR Method patient!

recommendations. (We'll discuss DMR Method research at greater length in the chapter entitled "DMR Method Research.")

Fourth, KARE 11, an NBC affiliate in Minneapolis, asked me to come have lunch with Dr. Mehmet Oz, star of the syndicated Dr. Oz Show, whose area of expertise is thoracic surgery. I was told that Dr. Oz wanted to hear about local health innovations from different providers while he was in town. In that meeting I explained the DMR Method, the research we were doing, and the amazing results we were seeing.

Dr. Oz told me that he had recently herniated a disc playing basketball and chose to treat it conservatively after receiving and rejecting a surgical recommendation from one of his peers. He was impressed with our research and with how our team was combining the best of physical therapy, chiropractic, rehabilitation, and conservative medical care to produce consistent results. He said he hoped that doctors and patients would become more aware of and try nonsurgical treatment options like he did before jumping straight to traditional medical management and surgery.

By the time I left that meeting with Dr. Oz, I realized that my team needed to produce a book—not only to educate healthcare providers and patients, but also to create a practical resource for patients to use while receiving treatment. Three years of nonstop collaboration and research later, you're holding the results of those efforts in your hands.

If You Are Considering Back Surgery

When Jim's doctor recommended surgery for his back condition, he rushed over to my office to question me about nonsurgical alternatives. I said, "Jim, I can't make any promises until I examine you, but more often than not, spinal conditions—even ones involving discs and nerves—can be helped through proper education, conservative treatment, and disciplined self-care." I also mentioned that the best neurosurgeons and orthopedic spine surgeons agree with that assessment and view surgery only as a last resort when all else has failed. After examining Jim and viewing his X-rays, I gave him the good news that he qualified for the DMR Method. His hopes for avoiding surgery increased even more when I told him that The DMR Method treatment protocol is backed by years of clinical case study research and that nineteen out of twenty cases from that research had been successfully treated without surgery.

If Jim's story is your story—spinal surgery has been recommended and you're searching for alternatives—rest assured that there's a good chance that the DMR Method can help you avoid surgery now and in the future.

If your doctor has recommended surgery for your spinal condition, consider these suggestions:

☐ *Read this book. It's designed to help you treat the underlying cause of your condition and teach you how to stay healthy and active. We know it works 96 percent of the time.*

☐ *Get an evaluation by a DMR Method provider. They are specially trained to identify when surgery is absolutely necessary and to create a customized comprehensive alternative care plan when surgery can be avoided. Before recommending surgery, many spine surgeons send their patients to us for evaluation because of the high success rate of the DMR Method.*

☐ *If surgery has been recommended, get a second opinion. If the second opinion varies wildly from the first opinion, get a third opinion.*

☐ *When seeking subsequent opinions, do not tell your new doctor what any previous doctors have recommended. If the new doctor's diagnosis and advice is different, then and only then should you share your previous doctors' recommendations with the new doctor.*

☐ *Don't agree to surgery because you're desperate for relief and want a quick fix. There are serious risks to consider.*

☐ *If your doctor recommends surgery, ask a lot of questions. Make sure you're fully informed about the risks, exactly what procedure is being recommended and why (especially if it's a fusion or appliance surgery), what you need to do before and after the surgery to ensure the best outcome, and what to expect during recovery and in the months and years to come.*

☐ *Find a surgeon who has been recommended by a trusted doctor or other healthcare provider. Your current medical provider may even be able to help you get an appointment with the recommended surgeon. It is not unusual to have to wait months before you can see a high-quality fellowship-trained surgeon.*

☐ *Avoid web-based services that ask you to send your scans to them for an opinion and recommendation. In-person interaction with your healthcare providers is essential.*

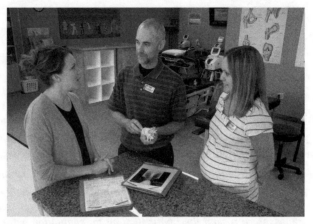

The DMR Method provides the right treatment in the right order to produce rapid, predictable and lasting results.

Fortunately, there are many excellent neurosurgeons and orthopedic spine surgeons to choose from who are both skilled and ethical. If and when surgery is indicated, a DMR Method provider's goal is to ensure that you are under the care of one of these surgeons. It may surprise you to learn that some of these surgeons have contributed essential knowledge, advice, and resources that have helped shape the DMR Method evaluation and treatment protocols. These highly regarded surgeons have also become one of the largest referral sources for the DMR Method.

The Promise of the DMR Method

The body has an amazing capacity to heal when obstacles to healing are removed. Too many back care programs focus only on treating symptoms or on strengthening muscles around the root cause of the problem, which can provide initial relief but ultimately stabilizes the dysfunction. Results are often disappointing and can worsen conditions until surgery is inevitable.

We learned from the first DMR Method clinical case study that combining elements of physical therapy, traction, chiropractic, and self-care makes all the difference. Each of those elements is crucial; if one is neglected, the patient's recovery will be compromised. For instance, while developing the DMR Method, physical therapists noticed that patients who were not getting skilled spinal manipulation from a chiropractor lagged behind in recovery.

Many patients who come to our center for treatment have done many of the right treatments but at the wrong time. Consequently, they are disappointed with the results. One common mistake was participating in a strengthening-based physical therapy program before addressing the underlying structural cause of the condition. Strengthening is important, but needs to be done at the right time and in the right sequence. The DMR Method provides the right treatment in the right order to produce rapid, predictable, and lasting results.

While I cannot guarantee results, I can tell you that 96.4 percent of the thousands of DMR Method patients we accept for care every year attain complete or significant relief from their symptoms, regain their ability to do the things they love to do, and completely avoid surgery.

The DMR Method was developed to end the confusion about back conditions and provide an effective and affordable treatment that offers lasting relief. Patients who have been suffering for years and have been through extensive treatment—sometimes even surgery—are shocked when I tell them that they are just a short time away from feeling better. If you or a loved one has been suffering from a herniated disc, sciatica, stenosis, slippage of a vertebrae, numbness or pain in your extremities, or chronic back and neck pain, I hope you find this book a useful resource in your healing journey.

Notes: _____

_____

_____

_____

_____

_____

_____

_____

_____

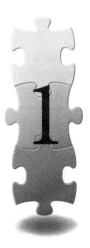

A Tour of Your Spine

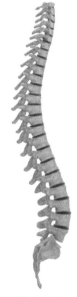

The spine is the most complex physical structure in the human body. It has the capacity to carry two to three times your body weight, it is flexible enough to allow you to bend and twist, and it provides the basic framework for the entire upper body. On the other hand, the spine can also be injured easily. Because the spine houses the spinal cord and is so tightly situated with all of the nerves that feed every muscle and organ in the entire body, any injury to the spine can result in considerable pain and disability, and can impair the function of other body systems as well.

Understanding the basic components and design of your spine, how closely it is associated with your nervous system, and the three pillars of body mechanics will help you better understand what can go wrong with the spine, why the DMR Method can be so effective in helping you recover, and how to avoid re-injury.

The Spine

The Basics of Bones, Joints, Muscles, and Nerves

Let's begin by talking about the overall framework of your body and how its four most important structural components—bones, joints, muscles, and nerves—work together to keep you mobile, properly aligned, and strong.

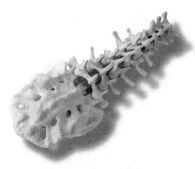

Lumbar Spine and Sacrum

The descriptions that follow apply to your entire body, but in the process you'll gain a better understanding of the amazing complexity of the spine.

Bones and Joints

The human skeleton is made up of more than two hundred bones that are connected by joints. Your bones are responsible for creating your body's general shape, and they serve to protect your internal organs and to manufacture blood cells. Each of your bones is made up of two compounds: a protein meshwork of collagen and a mineral form of calcium called hydroxyapatite.

The collagen fibers which make up the basic structure of your bones give them a great deal of resilience and make them resistant to breaking when twisted, bent, or impacted. It is actually the loss of this collagen meshwork and not just a loss of calcium that is responsible for the bone weakness associated with conditions such as osteoporosis. The other component of bone, hydroxyapatite, is a crystalline calcium salt which is integrated into the collagen meshwork. Hydroxyapatite is responsible for giving the bones rigidity as well as resistance to crushing under pressure.

Bones can be compared to steel-reinforced concrete; the collagen meshwork acts much like the steel meshwork in concrete and the hydroxyapatite acts much like the concrete surrounding the steel. Together they form a tough, resilient, and rigid framework upon which the rest of the body is supported. Since your bones are rigid and do not bend, you wouldn't be able to move if not for your joints.

Shoulder Joint

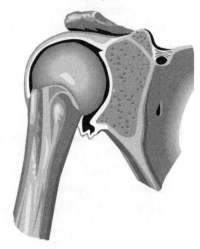

Joints are much more than simply a place where the ends of two bones meet. They are complicated systems of ligaments, tendons, membranes, and cartilage that allow the bones to move in a smooth, stable, and controlled way. Joints are designed in a variety of ways depending on their function and the particular stresses they have to endure. For example, the joints between your sternum (breastbone) and your ribs are simple joints consisting only of fibrous collagen. They're designed to be simple because the front part of your rib cage does not have to move very much in relation to your sternum. The shoulder joint, on the other hand, is an extremely complex joint that requires a whole host of muscles, ligaments, and tendons all working in concert with each other in order to move properly. If any one of the muscles or other structures of the shoulder are damaged, pain, instability, or loss of function may result.

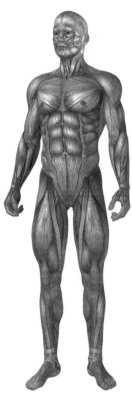

Muscles

There are more than six hundred fifty muscles in your body which have only one purpose: to create movement. While your bones are what give your body its framework, the muscles are what give your body motion. There are more than three times the number of muscles in your body as there are bones, and each one of these muscles fills a particular role in creating movement. Like bones, your muscles also contain a lot of collagen for strength and resilience. But instead of calcium salts, muscles contain a specialized type of cell which has the unique ability to contract when stimulated by the nervous system.

There are actually three types of muscle in the body: smooth muscle, cardiac muscle, and striated muscle (also called skeletal muscle). Smooth muscle is found surrounding the organs of the digestive tract as well as the arteries. In the digestive tract, smooth muscle is responsible for moving the food you eat through your digestive system, while the smooth muscle which surrounds the arteries helps the regulation of blood flow throughout the body. Unlike skeletal muscles, smooth muscles are involuntary muscles, meaning that you do not have conscious control over them.

Cardiac muscle, as its name implies, is found only in the heart. What differentiates cardiac muscle from all other muscle in the body is the fact that it rhythmically contracts on its own, regardless of stimulation by the nervous system. As a matter of fact, if two independent cardiac cells, each rhythmically contracting to their own beat, are put in contact with each other, they will begin beating in unison. That's a good thing, because otherwise your heart wouldn't beat very regularly.

Striated, or skeletal, muscle is the type of muscle that we can consciously control and that is of most interest to us because it is responsible for our posture and movement. Every skeletal muscle attaches to at least two different bones and, as they contract, they draw the bones together, using the joints as hinges, allowing controlled movement to take place.

Take, for example, the elbow joint. Compared to other joints in the body, such as the shoulder or hip, the elbow is a relatively simple hinge joint. Yet, there are more than a dozen muscles which cross the elbow joint, all of which contribute to the elbow's normal movement. If any of these muscles do not fire in a highly coordinated fashion, or if some of the muscles are tighter or weaker than they should be, abnormal joint function and pain may result. The spine is even more complex, with more than a hundred muscles that all have to fire in proper coordination in order for us to be able to walk, bend, lift, and even sit without experiencing pain.

The Nervous System

The nervous system consists of trillions of highly-specialized individual nerve cells, each of which communicates with hundreds or thousands of other nerve cells through tiny electrical pulses, and is comprised of two major systems. The central nervous system includes your brain and spinal cord; the peripheral nervous system includes the nerves that run from your spine to all areas of the body. The nervous system is called the master controller, as it is responsible for the control of all major body functions including our senses, movement, and balance, as well as the regulations of all bodily functions.

There are three types of nerves that are important to our discussion: pain nerves, motor nerves, and postural nerves. Pain nerves do just what their name implies—they allow you to feel pain. Whenever something in your body hurts, it's because the pain nerves in the area are being stimulated, sending signals to the brain to create the sensation of pain.

Motor nerves are responsible for controlling your movement by stimulating muscles to contract. You're able to hold this book in your hands because motor nerves are contracting the muscles in your hands and arms. If these nerves aren't able to function correctly, you may experience weakness, or even paralysis, in the muscles they control.

Postural nerves, or more correctly, proprioceptors, are sensory receptors that tell your brain where your body is in space. They are critical for proper balance, posture, and coordination—a process called proprioception. If you close your eyes and hold your arm out to your side, you can tell exactly where your arm is even though you can't see it because the proprioceptors in your arm and upper back tell your brain where your arm is.

If you've ever had too much to drink, you've experienced first-hand what happens when normal proprioception is disrupted. Alcohol interferes with the ability of your proprioceptors to communicate effectively with the area of your brain that's responsible for maintaining balance, posture, and coordination. That's why it becomes difficult to touch your finger to your nose when your eyes are closed, or to walk a straight line or stand up straight when you're intoxicated.

In the next section, we'll be pulling all of this information on bones, joints, muscles, and nerves together in a discussion about body mechanics.

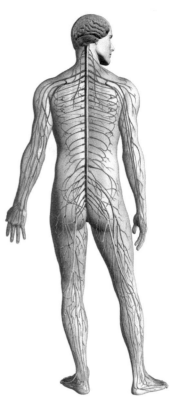

Understanding Your Spine

Your spine consists of nearly a hundred intricate joints connected together by a complicated meshwork of ligaments, tendons, cartilage, and muscles. The spine is designed to do three things simultaneously:

- to protect the spinal cord and the trillions of nerve pathways that serve as the primary communication conduit between your brain and the rest of your body;

- to serve as a structural support upon which all of your organs and upper body have to rest;

- to provide an incredible amount of mobility and flexibility, allowing you to bend forward to touch your toes, swim, throw a baseball, and turn your head. Unfortunately, with this degree of mobility and flexibility comes potential instability and the susceptibility to injury.

In order to function correctly, all of the bones, joints, muscles, and nerves have to work in perfect coordination. Any disruption in the position or movement in the bones of the spine, the loss of muscle balance, or a disruption in nervous coordination can lead to a host of problems, some of which will be discussed in the next chapter.

Fortunately, most of us don't experience severe problems with our spine or spinal cord, but small problems occur all the time. These happen when we slip and fall, are in a car accident, sleep in a strange bed, sit with poor

Spinal Nerves and Health

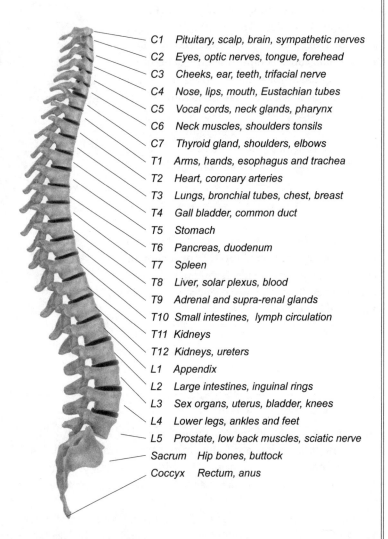

C1	Pituitary, scalp, brain, sympathetic nerves
C2	Eyes, optic nerves, tongue, forehead
C3	Cheeks, ear, teeth, trifacial nerve
C4	Nose, lips, mouth, Eustachian tubes
C5	Vocal cords, neck glands, pharynx
C6	Neck muscles, shoulders tonsils
C7	Thyroid gland, shoulders, elbows
T1	Arms, hands, esophagus and trachea
T2	Heart, coronary arteries
T3	Lungs, bronchial tubes, chest, breast
T4	Gall bladder, common duct
T5	Stomach
T6	Pancreas, duodenum
T7	Spleen
T8	Liver, solar plexus, blood
T9	Adrenal and supra-renal glands
T10	Small intestines, lymph circulation
T11	Kidneys
T12	Kidneys, ureters
L1	Appendix
L2	Large intestines, inguinal rings
L3	Sex organs, uterus, bladder, knees
L4	Lower legs, ankles and feet
L5	Prostate, low back muscles, sciatic nerve
Sacrum	Hip bones, buttock
Coccyx	Rectum, anus

Each of the nerves that exit the spine are connected to specific organs in the body. These nerves allow the brain to coordinate many bodily functions, such as digestion, heart rate, breathing, and many others. When these nerves become impinged, even slightly, the body's ability to regulate itself is impacted. This can lead to a variety of conditions, depending on which nerve is affected.

posture, "throw our back out," or lift something incorrectly. It's typically not just injury to the bones and joints themselves that causes misalignment in the spine. Damage to the muscles and connective tissue are just as important, for these are the structures that are responsible for supporting the bones and joints. Once these tissues are damaged, the vertebrae can lose their correct alignment or movement. That not only can cause pain and loss of function in the back, it can affect other areas of the body as well. Why? Damaged tissues can have an enormous impact on the intricate network of nerves emanating from the spine that are responsible for controlling and coordinating all the systems of your body.

The Construction of the Spine

The spine is made up of a stacked set of bones called the vertebrae, which are the "bricks" upon which our entire structure is built. Each vertebra consists of a vertebral body, which is a large oval-shaped solid block of bone, and a vertebral arch, which is located on the back of the vertebral body and creates the space through which the spinal cord runs.

Each vertebra is attached to two adjacent spinal vertebrae, with a disc between them. These discs, technically called intervertebral discs, are thick pads of fibrocartilage that act as shock absorbers and give the spine its ability to flex and twist. The disc itself is kind of like a jelly donut: it has an outer fibrous portion called the annulus, and a soft jelly-like center called the nucleus pulposus. Behind the disc and spinal cord are two smaller joints called facet joints, which are part of the vertebral arch; they help make your spine flexible and, along with the discs, bear the weight and stress that's put on the spine.

Between each pair of vertebrae and behind the disc is a small space where the nerves exit from the spinal cord and run to all the areas of the body. This space is called a vertebral foramen. Foramen is an impressive medical term that simply means "hole." Vertebral foramina (holes) can become compressed when a disc bulge or herniation presses into the area, inflammation causes the tissues in the area to swell, or if the intervertebral disc becomes dehydrated. When any of these things happen, excruciating pain can result; since the foramen is where you'll find nerves that control and coordinate most of the systems of your entire body, there can be far-reaching effects beyond the spine.

Ligaments bind the vertebrae together and tendons attach numerous muscles to each segment. These ligaments and tendons help absorb shock and restrict how much movement there is between each set of spinal vertebrae. Unfortunately, these ligaments and tendons can be damaged whenever spinal vertebrae are forcefully moved beyond their normal limits—such as in a whiplash or sports injury. An injury to a ligament is called a sprain. If the injury is to the tendon or muscle, it is referred to as a strain.

Muscles attach to the bony extensions of the vertebrae and provide movement in the spine by contracting in a highly coordinated way. Like ligaments, muscles are important for absorbing shock and releasing it in a controlled way. For example, when your heel strikes the ground as you walk, it is your muscles that lessen the shock before it reaches your head so that your teeth don't clatter together each time you take a step.

As a whole, the spine forms the protective housing for the spinal cord, which begins at the brain stem (back of the skull) and extends like a wire down the length of the spine. Ultimately, the spinal cord sends out nerve branches that send and receive signals from every cell in the body. The close relationship between the spine and the spinal cord means that damage or dysfunction to any of the vertebrae, discs, or supportive soft tissues can also affect the spinal cord or the nerves associated with it, causing pain or abnormal function of the structures innervated (supplied with nerves) by the affected area.

The Four Regions of the Spine

The spine is divided into four different regions. The upper seven vertebrae in the neck are collectively called the "cervical spine," with the skull sitting directly upon the first cervical vertebra (also called the Atlas). The middle twelve vertebrae are called the "thoracic vertebrae." All of the thoracic vertebrae have a pair of ribs attached to them. The twelve pairs of ribs are important for protecting several of your internal organs and are critical for breathing. The lower five vertebrae are referred to as the "lumbar vertebrae"; because they bear the full weight of your upper body, and are the most frequently injured. The lowest region of the spine is called the sacrum. In a young child, the sacrum is made up of five vertebrae, just like the lumbar spine. During later childhood, these five vertebrae fuse together to make one solid bone called the sacrum.

When viewed from the front or back, the spine should appear perfectly straight and symmetrical, reflecting the fact that your body is also symmetrical when viewed from the front or back. When viewed from the side, however, four major curves should be seen—one in each of the cervical, thoracic, lumbar, and sacral regions. In both the cervical and lumbar regions of the spine, the curves bend backward; these are called "lordotic" curves. The curves in the thoracic and sacral regions bend forward; these are called "kyphotic" curves. As strange as it may seem, these curves actually add a considerable amount

The Four Regions of the Spine

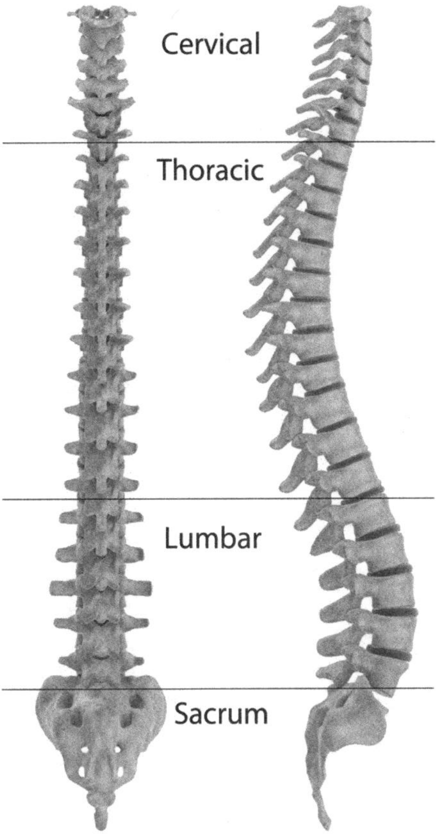

Cervical

Thoracic

Lumbar

Sacrum

There are four regions to the spine: the cervical, thoracic, lumber, and sacrum. The cervical and lumber regions are particularly prone to injury as they do not have supporting structures that the thoracic and sacrum regions have.

of strength and resiliency to the spine. Think about the curves as being like a spring, allowing the spine to flex and absorb shock much better than if it were straight. In fact, when a region of the spine loses its normal curve, as often happens in the neck following a whiplash injury, the discs that separate the vertebrae begin to degenerate.

Although the DMR Method principles of evaluation and treatment can be

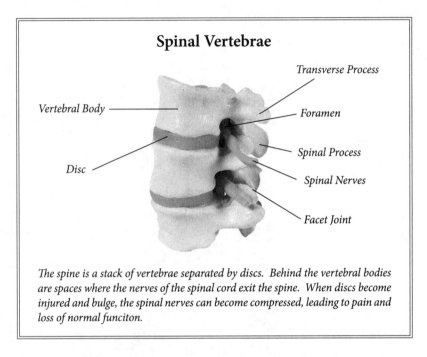

Spinal Vertebrae

Transverse Process

Vertebral Body

Foramen

Spinal Process

Disc

Spinal Nerves

Facet Joint

The spine is a stack of vertebrae separated by discs. Behind the vertebral bodies are spaces where the nerves of the spinal cord exit the spine. When discs become injured and bulge, the spinal nerves can become compressed, leading to pain and loss of normal funciton.

applied to any joint in the body, DMR Method practitioners end up working on the spine more than any other structure. That's because of the complexity and vulnerability of the spine and its potential for affecting so many systems of the body through its close association with the nervous system. Problems in the spine can come from a variety of sources:

- discs can become herniated and compress nerves that go to the legs or arms;
- the joints between the vertebrae may become stuck;
- the bones, ligaments, or joints themselves may be injured;
- the disc space itself can be a source of pain;
- the muscles surrounding the spine may become injured;
- muscle inflammation or spasm may develop due to overuse or injury;
- joint inflammation from overuse, injury, arthritis, or other disease.

The most common conditions that occur in the spine are described in the next chapter, "Understanding Your Condition."

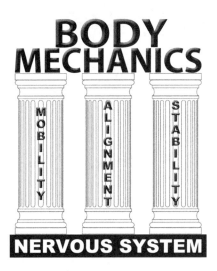

The Three Pillars Of Body Mechanics

The human body is an amazingly complex system of bones, joints, muscles, and nerves, all of which are designed to work together. The nervous system is the foundation, the master control system that integrates all the other systems of the body. When considering body mechanics, think of the nervous system as a network of wires that links your muscle, bones, and joints to your brain. Your brain sends out the right signals to control and coordinate how your body moves, but it's a two-way street. Your body is also continuously sending signals to your brain to help your brain create just the right signals to optimize how you control your body. Some of this control is voluntary and some is happening reflexively without you even knowing it. Assuming your nervous system is providing you with a solid foundation of control and coordination, there are three elements required to create balance and maximum efficiency in your body. We call them the three pillars of body mechanics.

The three pillars are Mobility, Alignment, and Stability. Understanding the importance of each and knowing how to effectively improve them and prevent their decline is paramount to the DMR Method. If you are lacking in any one of the pillars, your health will suffer. Not only does an imbalance in the three pillars cause pain and instability, it also has a devastating effect on your nervous system and your body's efficiency. Consequently, an imbalance can have far-reaching effects on your overall energy level, mental attitude, and even the internal systems of your body.

Consider a rowing team: all the parts of the boat and the bodies of the

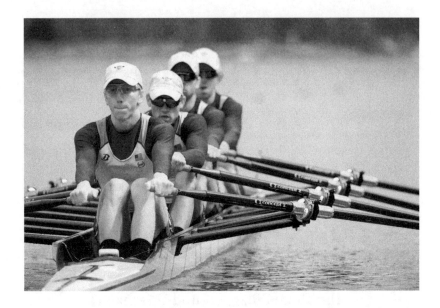

rowers have to be oriented properly to make the boat go in the right direction (Alignment). All the right parts of the boat and the rowers have to be move-able (Mobility). The rowers need a boat and bodies that are strong enough to hold up to stress and function properly (Stability). With all three of these elements in balance, the boat and rowers can glide through the water at a rapid clip. Any imbalance in the system will cause an immediate loss in effi-ciency and performance.

    If one of the oars locks up and stops moving (loss of Mobility), the rest of the team has to compensate to keep the boat from drifting off course. That creates an imbalance because some rowers have to compensate and exert more effort than others (loss of Alignment). The extra effort results in fatigue, and performance starts to suffer as the rowers struggle to stay on course (loss of Stability). The effects on performance are obvious when there's a breakdown in Mobility, Alignment, or Stability, but think about what else is going on. This situation will lead to excessive wear and tear on the boat and/or rowers that could make additional repairs necessary. It also couldn't help but affect the overall energy and attitude of the rowers. Clearly, just a little loss in mobility can set in motion a cascade of other events that can lead to pretty signifi-cant results. Let's spend a few moments discussing the three pillars of body mechanics individually.

Pillar One: Mobility

Over the years, I've had a number of patients with severe low-back pain who told me that their pain came on suddenly when they did something as simple as bend down to pet their cat, put on their socks, or take out the trash. Just about everyone would agree that a person's body should be able to handle such simple tasks. So what happened?

In every one of these cases, we found spinal joints that weren't moving properly; they were "all locked up." When the joints in one area of the spine don't move the way they should, other joints are forced to move more than they were designed to in an effort to compensate for the area that isn't moving. This causes undue stress and strain on the compensating joints and the muscles and ligaments surrounding them, which soon leads to pain and inflammation. At the same time, the areas that don't have normal movement will slowly worsen as the muscles continue to tighten, the joints become more dehydrated, and the ligaments and tendons shorten. This leaves the body in a very unstable state that, if left unchecked, will only worsen. Not only does good joint mobility decrease pain and disability, it's also essential for maintaining joint health. Motion is one of the key factors that helps your joints, including your discs, stay lubricated. That's why a person with arthritis can decrease disability and even slow the progression of their condition by safely maintaining as much motion as possible in the surrounding and affected joints. Joint mobility also stimulates the part of your nervous system that helps you maintain posture, alignment, and balance. Lack of motion in any joint shortcircuits this internal guidance system and makes you prone to alignment and stability issues.

As you will see later in this book, restoring joint mobility is the first step in the DMR Method treatment process. The maintenance of long-term

You Gotta Keep Movin'!

One morning a few years ago I had a patient who came in for a chiropractic visit and he was in a hurry. He had an exercise class at 10am, a lunch date at noon, bible study at 3 and a home association meeting at 7pm. After completing his treatment I grabbed my video camera and asked him to repeat his schedule for the day. When he was done I asked him one question, "Oliver, how old are you?" His answer, "98." I turned off the camera, looked at him and said, "That's awesome. You are my goal." He simply said, "Doc, you gotta keep movin'!"

mobility is essential for long-term management of spinal conditions. It will also help you stay active and age gracefully.

Pillar Two: Alignment

Your spine is designed to carry the weight of your body when it's in proper alignment. The natural arches from front to back in your neck, mid back, and lower back increase the strength of your spine. The joint angles, along with the distribution of weight between the two columns of facet joints and the larger column of vertebral body joints with discs between each, make the spine incredibly efficient and resilient—as long as it's in alignment. Proper alignment allows your bones to carry most of your weight with minimal stress on your muscles and ligaments. While muscles are well-suited for moving the body, they are not designed to carry the weight of the body. The moment your alignment varies from normal, your muscles have to work harder and your ligaments suffer more stress, even during normal physical activities.

Consider the dancer in the picture on the next page. Exceptional alignment and mobility is essential for her to produce and maintain her incredible pose. They enable her to achieve maximal efficiency in muscle strength and coordination with minimal stress on her body. Just a small curvature in her spine would cause her muscles to expend excessive energy to maintain her pose, which could severely affect her performance. Remember, proper spinal alignment allows your body to distribute stress efficiently on your skeleton and causes minimal stress on the muscles, ligaments, and discs between your vertebrae.

The most immediate problem with poor spinal alignment and posture is that it creates a lot of muscle compensation, fatigue, and overstressing. It also causes undue stress and strain on joints, discs, and supportive soft tissues, making them prone to aggravation and injury.

Optimal spinal alignment helps maximize muscle efficiency, decreases stress and strain on your spine, and drastically reduces your susceptibility to injury.

Pillar Three: Stability

The dancer pictured on the next page has amazing joint mobility and her alignment is optimal, but to achieve and maintain her pose she has to have equally impressive stability. Stability is achieved through strong, coordinated, and balanced muscles. Your muscles function much like the wires that hold up a tall radio or television antenna. If the wires are equally strong on all sides,

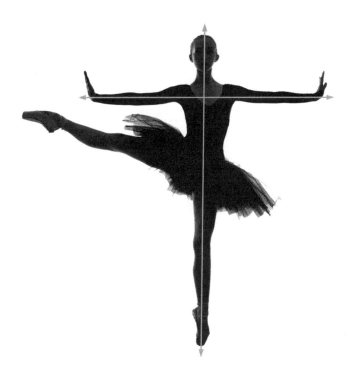

the antenna will stand up straight. If one of the wires becomes weak or breaks, the antenna will either lean to the side or collapse. The same is true with your body. If the muscles on all sides of your spine are balanced and strong, your body will stand up straight and strong.

Muscles get stronger or weaker in response to the demands placed on them. Since many of us sit at a desk, drive a car, and sit on the sofa at home, many of our muscles are not challenged. Consequently, they become weak. At the same time, the muscles that are constantly used throughout the day grow stronger. This imbalance of muscle strength contributes to poor posture and chronic muscle tension. Left unchecked, muscle imbalances tend to get worse, not better, because of a phenomenon called "reciprocal inhibition."

Reciprocal inhibition literally means "shutting down the opposite." Simply put, for all of the muscles that move your body in one direction, there are opposing muscles that move the body in the opposite direction. In order to keep these muscles from working against each other, when the body contracts one muscle group, it forces the opposing group to relax by essentially shutting down the opposite muscles. Consider people who work seated at a desk. Because all day long the muscles on the front side of the body are being used, the body essentially shuts down the opposite muscles in the upper back. Over

DMR Method™ Case Study
Severe Neck Pain Radiating into the Arm

Michael presented with severe neck pain rated 10/10 that radiated into his left shoulder and arm. The pain, which he described as sharp, was affecting his posture and severely limiting the mobility in his neck. He couldn't sleep comfortably and was awakened by pain multiple times during the night. His condition began fifteen years earlier after a car accident and had been progressively getting worse. No previous treatment had helped. His ability to be physically active had become extremely limited.

DIAGNOSIS

Following examination and imaging, he was diagnosed with multiple levels of cervical disc herniation, degenerative disc disease, severe subluxation (altered spinal alignment and mobility causing nerve irritation), and muscle spasm.

TREATMENT

The DMR Method chronic cervical protocol was prescribed with a focus on chiropractic adjustments (Integrated Progressive Mobilization), Dynamic Muscle Technique (DMT), cervical traction, and progressive exercise and stretching instruction to stabilize his recovery.

OUTCOME

Michael's symptoms completely resolved. His full range of motion was restored, and for the first time in years he could sleep though the night without being awakened by pain. He continues with his home exercise and stretching program, has resumed normal physical activity, and returns periodically for maintenance care.

DISCUSSION

This case underscores the tragic and degenerative effects of deficient mobility, alignment, and stability. It also demonstrates that coordinated care which focuses on the restoration of mobility, alignment, and stability (the three pillars of body mechanics) effectively decreases symptoms, stops progression of degeneration, and improves the quality of daily life.

time, the muscles in the upper back become weak. As we will see in the next section, this contributes to poor posture and chronic muscle spasms and pain.

The DMR Method starts by treating abnormal mobility and alignment and then stabilizing the correction with specific exercises to strengthen and balance the supporting muscles. Using proper body mechanics and following appropriate physical limitations is also essential to restoring stability. Stability helps make you balanced, strong, and resilient.

Pulling it All Together

Your spine is an incredibly complex and important structure for your overall health due to its close relationship to the spinal cord and nerves. If the spine is healthy, the central nervous system has the means with which to communicate and coordinate all of the body's functions. If there are any deficiencies in mobility, alignment, or stability, pain and disability can result. Any resulting interference to the nervous system can have far-reaching effects on all the systems and functions of your body. Focusing treatment on improving mobility, alignment, and stability not only causes a rapid decrease in symptoms and disability, it also prevents recurrence and helps your body and nervous system work at peak efficiency. Remember, in order to enjoy vibrant health, you have to make lifestyle choices that enhance rather than undermine your body's ability to be healthy. Treating spinal issues by restoring mobility, alignment, and stability is the core of the DMR Method evaluation and treatment process.

Notes:

_____

_____

_____

_____

_____

_____

_____

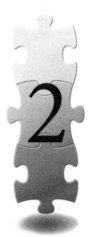

Understanding Your Condition

I vividly remember two things from an embryology class I had in graduate school. The first was the incredible complexity and mystical wonder of the development of the human body, and the second was why the health of the nervous system was so critical to normal development and well-being. Starting at conception, the body begins to take shape, beginning with the development of a long cylindrical tube that forms the spinal cord. From this cord, little bumps begin to form that make up all of the internal organs as well as the arms and legs. This process continues, seemingly by magic, for nine months until a fully formed human being emerges. As long as all of the organs function in a tightly controlled balance, the child will thrive and grow into a healthy adult.

The human body is amazing. While you calmly read this, your body is bristling with activity. The trillions of cells that make up your body are busy at work performing thousands of delicately balanced processes that support the miracle of life. The brilliance with which your body controls this profoundly complex dance of chemistry is breathtaking. As long as your body is able to keep "the dance" going, you remain healthy and vibrant. But any disruption in any of the body's processes can throw off the entire system and make you susceptible to disease.

The body's ability to regulate and control the synergistic balance of all of the necessary life processes is called "homeostasis." That term is derived from the Greek words for "same" and "steady." It refers to the way the body acts to maintain a stable internal balance. For example, your body works to maintain a carefully regulated internal temperature of 98.6 degrees. If you go outside on a warm day and begin to work, your body will begin to sweat in an effort to keep your temperature from rising too high. You may also begin to breathe deeper in an effort to keep your tissues supplied with oxygen during a period of increased demand.

The Three Forms of Stress

Physical
- Physical injuries
- Poor posture
- Repetative physical activity
- Over or under exercising

Biochemical
- Things we eat and drink
- The air we breath
- Anything we put on our skin

Psychological
- Our thoughts, feelings and emotions
- Not getting enough sleep

KEY POINT: All three forms of stress can contribute to the development of disease and disability. Effective treatment addresses each type of stress.

Disease and disability result whenever the body is stressed beyond its ability to maintain homeostasis. This stress comes in three forms; physical, biochemical, and psychological. See the chart above for examples of each form of stress. Understanding which forms of stress are causing or aggravating your condition and addressing each one of them appropriately is crucial to long-term and short-term recovery. DMR Method providers are specially trained to help you with this!

You are likely reading this book because you or a loved one is searching for a solution to a condition that has been causing pain and affecting the quality of daily life. Gaining clarity about the cause of your condition not only helps you understand the reasoning behind the steps in your recovery process, it can motivate you to consistently follow a self-care program.

Knowledge is power; the more you know about your condition the better. In this chapter, you'll find descriptions of many of the conditions we see regularly and treat successfully at DMR Method clinics. These conditions are organized into three categories; acute, chronic, and inherited (congenital).

Acute Conditions

Acute Lower Back Pain

Acute low-back pain (LBP) is pain that has been present for three months or less. It typically comes on quickly, usually following some kind of injury such as a slip and fall, lifting something heavy, or overtaxing underused muscles. The latter is often the cause of low-back pain among "weekend warriors"—people who engage in very little physical activity during the week, then push themselves way too much when the weekend arrives. By Sunday night, they are often flat on their backs.

The low back is a complicated structure of bones, joints, ligaments, and muscles that can easily be injured. You can sprain ligaments, strain muscles, damage discs, and irritate joints, all of which can lead to back pain. While sports injuries or accidents are more often the cause of acute low-back pain, sometimes even the simplest movements, like picking up a pencil from the floor, can have painful results.

Most cases of acute low-back pain will resolve through rest, ice, and conservative care. If your low-back pain is accompanied by radiating pain or numbness into your arms or legs, or if you notice changes in your bowel or bladder function, it's important to seek professional care immediately as such signs may indicate a serious problem.

Disc Herniation

You may have heard the term "slipped disc" used to describe a low-back injury. Discs do not actually "slip." Rather, they may herniate or bulge out from between the bones. A herniation is a displaced fragment of the center part or nucleus of the disc that is pushed through a tear in the outer layer (or annulus) of the disc. Pain results when irritating substances are released from this tear into surrounding tissues, and also if the fragment touches or compresses a nearby nerve. Disc herniation has some similarities to degenerative disc disease; in fact, discs that herniate are often in an early stage of degeneration. Herniated discs are common in the low back and neck.

A disc herniation starts with the internal shift of the nucleus (internal derangement), then the outer band around the disc tears (annular tear). Next, the nucleus begins to push outward and distort the outer band of the disc (disc prolapse) Then the nucleus breaks through the outer band and the nucleus oozes out of the disc (disc nucleus extrusion). The last stage of herniation occurs when a piece of the nucleus separates from the disc completely (disc sequestration).

The Progression of a Herniated Disc

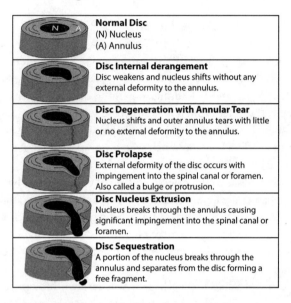

	Normal Disc (N) Nucleus (A) Annulus
	Disc Internal derangement Disc weakens and nucleus shifts without any external deformity to the annulus.
	Disc Degeneration with Annular Tear Nucleus shifts and outer annulus tears with little or no external deformity to the annulus.
	Disc Prolapse External deformity of the disc occurs with impingement into the spinal canal or foramen. Also called a bulge or protrusion.
	Disc Nucleus Extrusion Nucleus breaks through the annulus causing significant impingement into the spinal canal or foramen.
	Disc Sequestration A portion of the nucleus breaks through the annulus and separates from the disc forming a free fragment.

Amazingly, when a disc herniates it often doesn't cause any pain. Pain is typically caused by irritation of the nerves within the disc itself or by the disc herniation impinging upon a nerve that runs through the area.

The causes of disc herniation

Many factors decrease the strength and resiliency of the disc and increase the risk of disc herniation. Health-compromising lifestyle choices like smoking, lack of regular exercise, and inadequate nutrition can contribute to poor disc health. Poor posture, daily wear and tear, injury or trauma, and incorrect lifting or twisting can further stress the disc. Old injuries that have altered or weakened the supportive structures in the spine can also make a disc prone to herniation. As we age, our discs tend to dehydrate and break down. Often it's not just one factor that leads to a herniation, but rather the combination of different stressors that leads to the weakening of the disc. The disc may then herniate following a seemingly harmless movement like bending over to pick up a small object or even just coughing. Herniations are most common between the ages of thirty and forty because people in their thirties continue to be physically active while their body gradually becomes less resilient.

DMR Method Study

Pre-DMR Method MRI

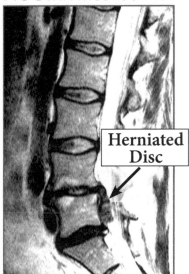

Herniated
Disc

Post-DMR Method MRI

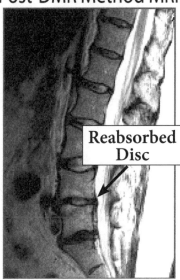

Reabsorbed
Disc

Massive Lumbar Disc Herniation Resolves

In the first photo, a massive disc herniation is visible that is impinging upon the spinal cord. Although this patient was unable to function and had pain radiating down their leg, they refused to consider spine surgery. They instead decided to try the DMR Method to see if that would help them. After two months of treatment with the DMR Method, the herniation is no longer visible and the patient's pain has dramatically improved. A seven year follow up revealed no recurrence of symptoms and normal functional abilities.

A severe herniation like this would normally be considered a surgical case. This is one of numerous case studies that demonstrate the remarkable healing capacity of the body when the proper therapeutic techniques are applied in the right order and at the right time. More information about this case and other case studies are in the DMR Research chapter.

Spinal Disc Herniation

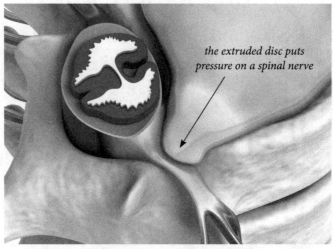

the extruded disc puts pressure on a spinal nerve

A disc herniation is a condition where damage to the outer structural fibers of the disc causes the disc to protrude, which can result in extreme pain and potential disability when the herniation puts pressure on a spinal nerve.

The symptoms of disc herniation

The most common symptom is pain in the area of the herniation. Depending upon the location of the herniation and the nerves it affects, you may experience radiating symptoms of pain and/or numbness in the distribution of the nerves. In low-back herniations, the hips and legs are most affected; in neck herniations, the shoulders and arms are most affected. In severe cases of disc herniations, weakness can develop in the affected extremity and you can experience changes in bowel or bladder habits and may have difficulty with sexual function. These severe cases may lead to medical emergencies.

Sciatica

The sciatic nerve is the longest nerve in your body. It runs from your pelvis, through your hip area and buttocks, and down each leg. The sciatic nerve branches into smaller nerves as it travels down the legs, providing feeling to your thighs, legs, and feet as well as controlling many of the muscles in your lower legs. The term sciatica refers to pain that radiates along the path of this nerve, which may be caused by any number of conditions.

BIG IDEA! Bend and Twist — Injure Your Disc!

When it comes to the health of your spinal discs, the single-worst thing you can do is to twist your back while bent over. The combination of bending and twisting places extraordinary stress on the disc and makes it very susceptible to injury. Unfortunately, it is sometimes difficult to avoid bending and twisting because so many daily activities require it, such as shoveling snow, placing groceries into your car, lifting objects off the floor that are located behind other objects, and even putting on your shoes. There are techniques that you can use to minimize the stress on the low back, which will be discussed in the Lifestyle and Exercise Guide towards the end of this book..

The most common cause of sciatica is compression from a herniated lumbar disc. Other conditions that can causes sciatica include:

- Lumbar spinal stenosis. Your spinal cord is a bundle of nerves that extends the length of your spine. It's housed inside a channel (spinal canal) within the vertebrae. Thirty-one pairs of nerves branch off from the spinal cord, providing communication between your brain and the rest of your body. In spinal stenosis, one or more areas in the spinal canal or the openings between the vertebrae narrow, putting pressure on the spinal cord or on the roots of these branching nerves. When the narrowing occurs in the lower spine, the lumbar and sacral nerve roots may be affected.

- Spondylolisthesis. This condition, often the result of degenerative disc disease, occurs when one vertebra slips slightly forward over another vertebra. The displaced bone may pinch a portion of the sciatic nerve where it leaves the spine.

- Piriformis syndrome. Running directly above the sciatic nerve, the piriformis muscle starts at your lower spine and connects to each thigh bone (femur). Piriformis syndrome occurs when the muscle becomes tight or goes into spasms, putting pressure on the sciatic nerve. Active women—runners and serious walkers, for example—are especially prone to develop the condition. Prolonged sitting, car accidents, and falls also may contribute to piriformis syndrome.

- Spinal tumors. A tumor is a mass of abnormal cells. In the spine, these growths may occur inside the spinal cord within the membranes (meninges) that cover the spinal cord, or in the space between the spinal cord and the vertebrae—the most common site. As it grows, a tumor compresses the cord itself or the nerve roots. This compression can cause severe back pain that may extend to your hips, legs, or feet; muscle weakness and a loss of sensation — especially in your legs; difficulty walking; and sometimes loss of bladder or bowel function.

- Trauma. A car accident, fall, or blow to the spine can injure the lumbar or sacral nerve roots.

- Sciatic nerve tumor or injury. Although uncommon, the sciatic nerve itself may be affected by a tumor or injury, leading to sciatic pain.

- Other causes. In some cases, your doctor may not be able to find a cause for your sciatica. A number of problems can affect the bones, joints, and muscles, all of which could potentially result in sciatic pain.

How do you know if you have sciatica?

Pain that radiates from your lower (lumbar) spine to your buttock and down the back of your leg is the hallmark of sciatica. Sciatica may be accompanied by numbness, tingling, and muscle weakness in the affected leg. This pain can vary widely, from a mild ache to a sharp, burning sensation or excruciating discomfort. Sometimes it may feel like a jolt or electric shock. Sciatic pain often starts gradually and intensifies over time. It's likely to be worse when you sit, cough, or sneeze. Usually only one lower extremity is affected, but you may feel the discomfort almost anywhere along the nerve pathway. It's especially likely to follow one of these routes:

- from your lower back to your knee;

- from the mid-buttock to the outside of your calf, the top of your foot, and into the space between your last two toes;

- from the inside of your calf to your inner ankle and sole.

In addition to pain, you may also experience:

- Numbness or muscle weakness along the nerve pathway in your leg or foot. In some cases, you may have pain in one part of your leg and numbness in another.

- Tingling or a pins-and-needles feeling. This occurs most commonly in your toes or part of your foot.

- A loss of bladder or bowel control. This is a sign of cauda equina syndrome, a rare but serious condition that requires emergency care. If you experience either of these symptoms, seek medical help immediately.

Facet Syndrome

The facet joints connect the posterior elements of the vertebrae to one another. Like the bones that form other joints in the human body, such as the hip, knee, or elbow, the surfaces of the joints are covered by a layer of smooth cartilage, surrounded by a capsule of ligaments, and lubricated by synovial fluid. Just like other joints, the facet joints can become inflamed and painful when injured or over-stressed. The hallmark symptom of facet syndrome is local sharp pain that can makes it difficult to change positions or stand up straight.

If not treated properly, facet syndrome can lead to a chronic degenerative condition called facet arthropathy, a form of arthritis that affects the facet joints of the spine. Although joints affected by facet arthropathy are typically not as painful as they are during an episode of facet syndrome, significant damage may occur to the joint surfaces over time that can lead to long-term loss of motion and weakness.

Acute Neck Pain

Almost everyone has experienced acute neck pain at some point. It can come on suddenly or develop slowly over time. It can be the result of an injury, chronic poor posture, sleeping the wrong way, or can even be brought

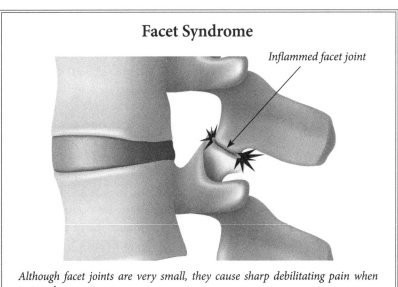

Facet Syndrome

Inflammed facet joint

Although facet joints are very small, they cause sharp debilitating pain when irritated.

on by excessive emotional stress. In addition to causing local neck pain and stiffness, it can radiate into the upper back and shoulders, or cause headaches that start at the base of the skull and radiate all the way into the forehead.

Acute neck pain that lasts for more than two days should be evaluated and treated appropriately to prevent it from developing into something worse. Most cases of acute neck pain will resolve through rest, ice, gentle stretching, and conservative care. If your neck pain is accompanied by radiating pain or numbness into your arms, or if you experience dizziness or light-headedness, seek professional care immediately as these symptoms may indicate a serious problem.

Whiplash Injury

Whiplash is by far the most common type of neck injury. Whiplash is caused by a sudden movement of the head— backward, forward, or sideways— that results in the damage to the supporting muscles, ligaments, and other connective tissues in the neck and upper back. Whether from a car accident, sports, or an accident at work, whiplash injuries must be taken seriously. Given that symptoms of a whiplash injury can take weeks or months to manifest, it is easy to be fooled into thinking that you are not as injured as you really are.

People often don't seek treatment following a car accident or sports-related whiplash injury because they experience little or no immediate pain. Unfortunately, by the time more serious complications develop, damage done by the injury may have become permanent. Numerous studies have shown that years after a person has sustained a whiplash injury, roughly half of them state that they still suffer with symptoms from their injuries. If you have been in a motor vehicle or any other kind of accident, please don't assume that you escaped injury simply because you are not currently experiencing pain. DMR Method practitioners can perform a simple evaluation to determine if you have any injuries that require treatment. If proper clinical and self-care treatment is done right away, you are more likely to recover rapidly and avoid permanent damage.

There are four distinct phases that occur during a whiplash injury while your body is experiencing an extremely rapid and intense acceleration and deceleration. In fact, all four phases of a whiplash injury occur in less than one-half of a second! At each phase, there is a different force acting on the body that contributes to the overall injury, and with such a sudden and forceful movement, damage to the vertebrae, nerves, discs, muscles, and ligaments of your neck and spine can be substantial.

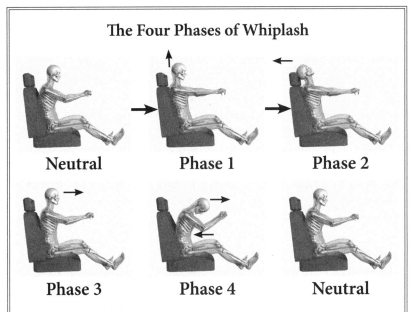

The Four Phases of Whiplash

Neutral   **Phase 1**   **Phase 2**

Phase 3   **Phase 4**   **Neutral**

In phase 1, the seat pushes against the mid-back causing an upward compression force in the neck. While it is still compressed, the neck is rapidly forced backward and forward in phases 2-4, resulting in damage to the discs, muscles, and connective tissues.

Injuries Resulting from Whiplash Trauma

Whiplash injuries can manifest in a wide variety of ways, including neck pain, headaches, fatigue, upper back and shoulder pain, cognitive changes, and low-back pain. Due to the fact that numerous factors—including direction of impact, speed of the vehicles involved, sex, age, and physical condition—contribute to the overall whiplash trauma, it's impossible to predict the pattern of symptoms that each individual will suffer. Additionally, whiplash symptoms commonly have a delayed onset, often taking weeks or months to present. There are, however, a number of conditions that health providers commonly see.

Neck pain

Neck pain is the single most common complaint resulting from whiplash trauma, reported by over 90 percent of patients. Typically, this pain radiates across the shoulders, up into the head, and down between the shoulder blades.

Whiplash injuries tend to affect all of the tissues in the neck, including the facet joints and discs between the vertebrae as well as all of the muscles, ligaments, and nerves.

Facet joint pain is the most common cause of neck pain following a car accident. Facet joint pain is typically felt on the back of the neck, just to the right or left of center, and is usually tender to the touch. Facet joint pain, which cannot be visualized on X-rays or MRIs, can only be diagnosed by physical palpation of the area.

Disc injury is also a common cause of neck pain, especially chronic pain. The outer wall of the disc (called the annulus) is made up of bundles of fibers that can be torn during a whiplash trauma. These tears can lead to disc degeneration or herniation, resulting in irritation or compression of the nerves running through the area. This irritation or compression commonly causes pain to radiate into the arms, shoulders, and upper back, and may result in muscle weakness.

Damage to the muscles and ligaments in the neck and upper back are the major cause of the pain experienced in the first few weeks following a whiplash injury, and is the main reason why patients experience stiffness and restricted range of motion. Damage to the ligaments often results in abnormal movement and instability.

Headaches

After neck pain, headaches are the most prevalent complaint among those suffering from whiplash injury, affecting more than 80 percent of all people. While some headaches are actually the result of direct brain injury, most are related to injury of the muscles, ligaments, and facet joints of the cervical spine, which refer pain to the head. That's why treating the supporting structures of the patient's neck is such an important step in alleviating a patient's headaches.

BIG IDEA! Treat Whiplash Injuries Immediately!

Most whiplash injuries can be treated successfully in 8-12 weeks if a person seeks immediate attention for their injuries. If that same person waits a few weeks or months before seeking treatment, they can be looking at months of treatment, and the likelihood of them never fully recovering increases greatly. If you have sustained a whiplash injury, Early intervention is the key!

TMJ problems

A less common, but very debilitating disorder that can result from whip-lash is temporomandibular joint dysfunction (TMJ). TMJ usually manifests as pain together with clicking and popping noises in the jaw during movement. If not properly evaluated and treated, TMJ problems can continue to worsen and lead to headaches, facial pain, ear pain, and difficulty in eating.

Brain injury

A mild to moderate brain injury can occur during a whiplash injury, due to the forces impacting the brain during the four phases mentioned earlier. The human brain is a soft structure, suspended in a watery fluid called cere-brospinal fluid. When the brain is forced forward and backward in the skull, the brain bounces off the inside of the skull, which can lead to bruising or bleeding in the brain itself. In some cases, patients temporarily lose conscious-ness and have symptoms of a mild concussion. More often, even though there is no loss of consciousness, patients complain of mild confusion or disorienta-tion just after the crash. The long-term consequences of a mild brain injury can include mild confusion, difficulty concentrating, sleep disturbances, irri-tability, forgetfulness, loss of sex drive, depression, and emotional instability. Although less common, the nerves responsible for your sense of smell, taste, and even your vision may be affected as well, resulting in a muted sense of taste, changes in your sensation of smell, and visual disturbances.

Low-back pain

Although most people consider whiplash to be an injury of the neck, the low back is also commonly injured. In fact, low-back pain is found in more than half of rear-impact collisions in which injury was reported, and almost three-quarters of all side-impact crashes. This is mostly due to the fact that the low back experiences a tremendous compression during the first two phases of a whiplash injury, even though it does not approach the degree of flexion-extension injury experienced in the neck.

Thoracic Outlet Syndrome

Thoracic outlet syndrome (TOS) occurs when the network of blood vessels and nerves (brachial plexus) that exit from the lower neck becomes compressed in the space between your collarbone and your first rib (thoracic

Thoracic Outlet Syndrome

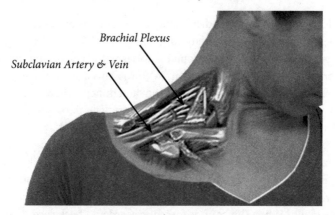

Brachial Plexus

Subclavian Artery & Vein

outlet). This can lead to significant pain, tingling, or weakness in your neck, shoulder, arm, hand, or fingers. Although some cases of TOS may eventually resolve over time on their own, the condition can gradually become worse and lead to significant long-term problems if left untreated.

Thoracic outlet syndrome is often caused by some form of physical trauma, such as a severe fall, auto accident, or sports injury, or from the repetitive occupational stress resulting from poor ergonomics in the workplace. Certain anatomical differences may increase the likelihood of developing TOS; for example, women tend to have smaller thoracic outlet openings than men, as well as cervical ribs that may impinge on the thoracic outlet. Regardless of the cause, most cases of TOS respond well to the DMR Method treatment.

Subluxation
The Link Between Acute and Chronic Spinal Conditions

A number of acute conditions can affect the spine, many of which turn into more serious or chronic conditions due to two words: vertebral subluxation. Subluxation refers to any alteration in a joint's mobility or alignment that affects the ability of the joint to function normally.

Subluxation is typically caused by traumatic or repetitive use injuries, poor posture, lack of exercise, or some combination of these factors. Nutrition, stress, and genetic predisposition can also play a role. Subluxations can cause irritation to the local nerves as well as the nerves that emanate from the spine to supply other areas of the body. If subluxations are not addressed properly, an acute injury like whiplash or a disc herniation can result in residual joint mobility and alignment issues. Over time, these effects can lead

Lower Back (Lumbar) Subluxation

to additional wear and tear to the joint and supportive soft tissues, resulting in joint inflammation, scar tissue formation, and imbalanced muscles and ligaments. Any one of these issues can trigger local pain and dysfunction as well as pain and dysfunction in other areas.

Consider a person who has a subluxation (altered mobility and alignment) in the lower back as the result of a sports injury. The imbalance causes the right gluteal muscle to contract more than the left, which can irritate the sciatic nerve and radiate pain into the leg (see illustration below). Healthcare providers could treat the gluteal muscle to alleviate pressure on the sciatic nerve, but if they don't treat the subluxation imbalance in the spine the condition will recur. Over time, the patient's symptoms and attendant pain may worsen and make the patient prone to other conditions such as disc herniation.

Identifying and correcting vertebral subluxation is an essential element in treating both acute and chronic conditions. The earlier that vertebral subluxation is detected, the better the chance of preventing an acute condition from developing into something more serious and chronic.

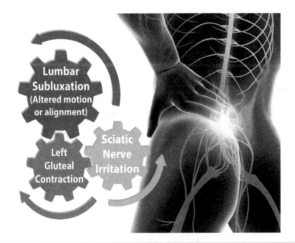

The DMR Method definition of Subluxation

A subluxation is altered mobility or alignment of a joint that alters the normal mechanical function of the joint. It causes an imbalance in the nerves that control and coordinate local joint function, and can also cause imbalance in associated nerves that control and coordinate other areas of the body.

Chronic Conditions

Degenerative Disc Disease (DDD)

Degenerative disc disease is a common syndrome usually involving an initial injury to a disc and the progressive degenerative changes that follow. Discs are pads that separate the vertebrae. Each disc consists of a ring of tough fibrous tissue (annulus fibrosis) surrounding a soft, gel-like center (nucleus pulposus) and a thin pad of cartilage on the top and bottom of each disc (cartilagenous end-plates). The blood supply to the disc is only to the cartilagenous end-plates. The part of the disc that doesn't receive a direct blood supply uses a "pump mechanism" to absorb fluid and stay hydrated. Disc degeneration begins when this pump mechanism stops working efficiently. As a disc deteriorates, the tough, outer layer becomes brittle and tears easily with minor stress or trauma. At the same time, the jelly-like center starts to dry out. As this happens, the entire disc spreads out (bulges) and shrinks in height.

With DDD you may not experience any pain or dysfunction until you bend or twist the "wrong" way one day. This causes the disc to tear further and release inflammatory substances into the surrounding tissue, which causes nerve irritation and results in low-back pain. In DDD, the combination of instability and tissue inflammation results in mild to severe chronic low-back pain and stiffness that can be mild or severe. If the DDD is also causing

The Progression of Degenerative Disc Disease

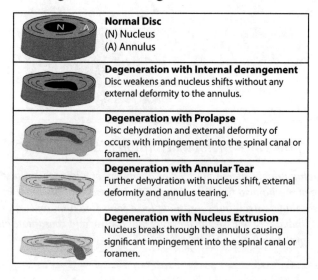

Normal Disc
(N) Nucleus
(A) Annulus

Degeneration with Internal derangement
Disc weakens and nucleus shifts without any external deformity to the annulus.

Degeneration with Prolapse
Disc dehydration and external deformity of occurs with impingement into the spinal canal or foramen.

Degeneration with Annular Tear
Further dehydration with nucleus shift, external deformity and annulus tearing.

Degeneration with Nucleus Extrusion
Nucleus breaks through the annulus causing significant impingement into the spinal canal or foramen.

compression of a nerve root, the pain may radiate down the legs or into the feet, and may be associated with numbness and tingling or weakness in these areas.

It is difficult if not impossible to diagnose DDD without an X-ray or MRI. If degenerative disc disease is present, X-rays will often show a narrowing of the spaces between the vertebrae, which indicates that the disc has become too thin or has collapsed.

Spinal Stenosis

In spinal stenosis, narrowing occurs in the "tunnels" or holes that the spinal cord or spinal nerve roots travel through—the spinal canal and the intervertebral foramen. When the nerves do not have enough room, they are compressed by the bony structures around them. When nerves are compressed, they respond by sending pain signals to the brain.

Spinal stenosis may be caused by anything that decreases the size of your spinal canal or intervertebral foramen. You may have been born with an abnormally small spinal canal or intervertebral foramen or these holes may become narrowed through the process of degenerative changes. Shrinkage of the discs, formation of bone spurs, and thickening of surrounding ligaments may all result in less space through which the nerves may travel.

Some people with spinal stenosis are symptom-free or only experience occasional mild pain in their low back. Others have symptoms that are so severe that they cannot even walk. If you have significant spinal stenosis, you will notice pain in your low back, buttocks, thighs, or legs that gets worse with standing or walking, and improves with rest. You may also have numbness, tingling, and weakness in the lower extremities.

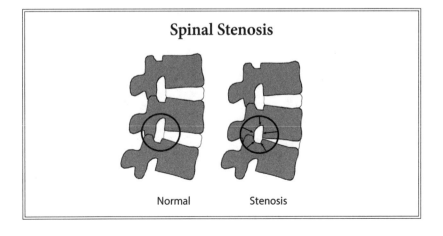

Spinal Stenosis

Normal   Stenosis

Spondylolisthesis

The term "spondylolisthesis" simply means that one vertebra has slipped forward on the vertebra below it. In order for this to happen, a part of the vertebrae called the "pars interarticularis" is either malformed or has been fractured at some point. There are two types of spondylolisthesis: congenital and acquired. If you have congenital spondylolisthesis, you were likely born with this condition, though symptoms are usually not experienced until later in childhood or even adulthood. Acquired spondylolisthesis occurs later in life. It may be degenerative, occurring due to the daily cumulative stresses you put on your spine, or it may occur following trauma. Spondylolisthesis is much more common in physically active people. Fully half of those with spondylolisthesis recall some sort of injury prior to developing pain.

People with either type of spondylolisthesis are often nonsymptomatic. X-rays will show if you have this condition. Those experiencing symptoms typically experience pain with movement and during recovery after extended periods of physical activity. You may have tight hamstring muscles or may notice that you have "swayback," which is an increased lumbar curve (lordosis). As spondylolisthesis worsens, patients often experience progressively disabling pain and disability upon waking in the morning.

Since spondylolisthesis can be progressive and worsen with time, taking action with appropriate treatment is essential, even if you haven't experienced any symptoms after being diagnosed.

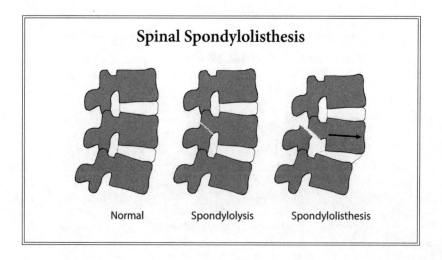

Spinal Spondylolisthesis

Normal   Spondylolysis   Spondylolisthesis

Spondylolisthesis Success!

Diane was disabled with spondylolisthesis. Every morning she had severe back pain and immobility. It took her several hours to get up and moving. She was very limited in her ability to any physical activity without increasing her pain and the quality of her life was poor. She was contemplating surgery when she heard about the DMR Method.

After a thorough evaluation, she followed a DMR Method protocol that was specifically designed for spondylolisthesis. Progress was slow at first, but with consistent clinical care and strict adherence to restrictions, home exercises, stretches and use of proper body mechanics her condition dramatically improved. She now gets out of bed pain free and enjoys an active lifestyle including daily workouts, snowmobiling and grandkid activities. Diane is a testament to the benefits of following all of the elements of the DMR Method.

Headaches

Headaches, which affect just about everyone at some point, can present themselves in many different ways. Some people only experience pain in one part of their head or behind their eyes; some people experience a pounding sensation inside their entire head; and some people experience nausea. The pain itself may be dull or sharp and may last for anywhere from a few minutes to a few days. Fortunately, very few headaches have serious underlying causes, but those that do require urgent medical attention.

Headaches can be due to a wide variety of causes, including drug reactions, temporomandibular joint dysfunction (TMJ), tightness in the neck muscles, low blood sugar, high blood pressure, stress, and fatigue. The majority of recurrent headaches are either tension headaches (also called cervicogenic headaches) or migraine headaches. A third, less common, type, known as a cluster headache, is a cousin to the migraine. Let's take a brief look at each of these types.

Tension Headaches

Tension headaches are the most common, affecting upwards of 75 percent of all headache sufferers. Most people describe a tension headache as a constant dull, achy feeling, as if there were a tight band around their head or behind their eyes. These headaches usually begin slowly and gradually, most often in the middle of or toward the end of the day. Tension headaches are often the result of stress or bad posture, which stresses the spine and muscles in the upper back and neck.

Tension headaches rarely last more than several days, but in some cases may persist for many months. Although the pain can at times be severe, tension headaches are usually not associated with symptoms such as nausea, throbbing sensations, or vomiting.

The most common cause of tension headaches is subluxations in the upper back and neck—especially the upper neck. Subluxations are alterations in the mobility and alignment of a joint that cause irritation to the associated nerves. Subluxations often have trigger points associated with them. A trigger point is a type of "knot" in the muscle that is painful when pressed and often causes referred pain. When the top cervical vertebrae lose their normal motion or position, a small muscle called the rectus capitis posterior minor (RCPM) muscle goes into spasm. This small muscle has a tendon which slips between the upper neck and the base of the skull and attaches to a thin tissue called the dura mater that covers the brain. Although the brain itself has no feeling, the dura mater is very pain-sensitive. Consequently, when the RCPM muscle goes into spasm and its tendon tugs at the dura mater, a headache results.

Another cause of tension headaches comes from referred pain from trigger points in the Sternocleidomastoid (SCM) or levator muscle on the side of the neck. These are common in people who suffer a whiplash injury due to the muscle damage in the neck region.

Migraine Headaches

Each year, about 25 million people in the U.S. experience migraine headaches; about 75 percent of those suffering from migraines are women. Migraines are intense, throbbing headaches that are often associated with nausea and sensitivity to light or noise. They can last from a few hours to a few days. Many who suffer from migraines experience visual symptoms called an "aura" just prior to an attack. This aura is often described as "seeing flashing lights"; others report that everything takes on a dream-like appearance.

Migraine sufferers usually have their first attack before age thirty. Migraines often run in families, supporting the notion that they have a genetic component. Some people have attacks several times a month; others have less than one a year. Most people find that migraine attacks occur less frequently and become less severe as they get older.

Migraine headaches are caused by a constriction of the blood vessels in the brain, followed by a dilation of blood vessels. During the constriction of the blood vessels, a decrease in blood flow leads to the visual symptoms experienced by many. Most people who don't experience the classic migraine aura can also sense that an attack is imminent. Once the blood vessels dilate, a rapid increase in blood pressure inside the head leads to the pounding headache. Each time the heart beats, another shock wave is sent through the carotid arteries in the neck up into the brain.

There are many theories about why the blood vessels constrict in the first place, but no one knows for sure. What we do know is that there are a number of things that can trigger migraines, such as lack of sleep, stress, flickering

---

DMR Method Case Study - Migraine Headaches

HISTORY

Nicole had issues with severe migraines her entire life. Sitting created a lot of tension and pain in her neck and upper back, and even into her right shoulder at times. Her migraines significantly affected her job and personal life. She missed work on a regular basis and took prescription medication for pain and migraines.

DIAGNOSIS

An X-ray exam revealed mild scoliosis of Nicole's cervical spine and forward head posture. DMR Method Evaluation revealed severe fixation/subluxation of the upper cervical spine and upper thoracic spine. Nicole also experienced extensive muscle spasm as well as ligament and joint capsule restriction.

TREATMENT

Treatment included the Chronic DMR Method protocol with a focus on Integrative Progressive Manipulation (IPM) and Dynamic Muscle Technique (DMT). A cervical extension wedge was prescribed for home use.

OUTCOME

Nicole's migraines were completely alleviated. Four months later, Nicole stated, "This is the best I have ever felt." She has resumed all normal physical activity and no longer misses work due to migraines.

lights, strong odors, changing weather patterns, and several foods—especially foods that are high in an amino acid called tyramine.

Cluster Headaches

Cluster headaches are typically short-duration, excruciating headaches, usually felt on one side of the head behind the eyes. Cluster headaches affect about one million people in the U.S. Unlike migraines, cluster headaches are more common in men. This is the only type of headache that tends to occur at night. They're called "cluster" headaches because they tend to occur one to four times per day over a period of several days. After one cluster of headaches is over, it may be months or even years before they occur again. Like migraines, cluster headaches are likely to be related to a dilation of the blood vessels in the brain, causing a localized increase in pressure.

Fibromyalgia

The word fibromyalgia comes from the Latin term for fibrous tissue (fibro) and the Greek terms for muscle (myo) and pain (algia). Fibromyalgia syndrome is a chronic disorder of widespread muscle pain, fatigue, and multiple tender points that affects three to six million people in the U.S. For reasons that are yet unclear, more than 90 percent of those who develop fibromyalgia are women. This may be due to the socialization of women in American culture or it may be attributed to female reproductive hormones and other genetic predispositions.

According to the American College of Rheumatology (ACR), fibromyalgia is defined as a history of pain in all four quadrants of the body lasting more than three months. Pain in all four quadrants means that you have pain in both your right and left sides, as well as above and below the waist. The ACR also described eighteen characteristic tender points on the body associated with fibromyalgia. In order to be diagnosed with fibromyalgia, a person must have eleven or more of these tender points (see illustration on the next page). In addition to pain and fatigue, people who have fibromyalgia may experience:

- Sleep disturbances
- Morning stiffness
- Headaches
- Irritable bowel syndrome

- Painful menstrual periods

- Numbness or tingling of the extremities

- Restless legs syndrome

- Temperature sensitivity

- Cognitive and memory problems (sometimes referred to as "fibro fog")

Fibromyalgia is often confused with another condition called "myofascial pain syndrome" or "myofascitis." Both fibromyalgia and myofascitis can cause pain in all four quadrants of the body and tend to have similar tender point locations, but the two conditions are worlds apart. Myofascitis is an inflammatory condition due to overuse of or injury to your muscles, whereas fibromyalgia is a chronic condition that involves disrupted hormones and tissue repair. Whereas myofascitis tends to come on rather suddenly and is usually associated with a particular activity or injury, fibromyalgia has a slow, insidious onset, usually beginning in early adulthood. It is important to diagnose each of these correctly, for they require different approaches to treatment. Unfortunately, fibromyalgia is a chronic condition, meaning it lasts a long time—possibly a lifetime. The good news is that it won't cause damage to your joints, muscles, or internal organs.

Some research suggests that fibromyalgia may be a form of stress-related condition that is a cousin to systemic lupus erythematosus (often referred to as simply "lupus") and chronic fatigue syndrome. All three conditions affect mostly women and include chronic fatigue, sleep disturbances, irritable

Fibromyalgia Pain Points

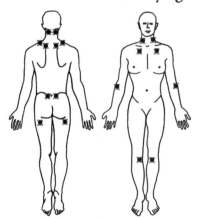

Those with fibromyalgia tend to display tenderness in 18 different points on the body. A diagnosis of fibromyalgia requires tenderness in at least 11 of these 18 points and at least one tender point in all four quadrants of the body.

bowel, and other similarities. Think of these three conditions as a continuum with fibromyalgia on one end, lupus on the other end, and chronic fatigue syndrome in the middle. All three are caused by an abnormal stress response in the body, but with lupus, the immune system is primarily affected, causing an autoimmune reaction that attacks your healthy tissues. On the other end of the spectrum is fibromyalgia, in which metabolic abnormalities are primary. These metabolic changes are the result of a stress-induced decrease in blood flow to an area of the brain called the pituitary. This in turn causes a decrease in a number of important hormones, such as "growth hormone releasing hormone" (GHRH or somatotropin) and "thyroid stimulating hormone." These hormonal changes lead to abnormal muscle healing, borderline or full-blown hypothyroid, and memory and cognitive changes.

One of the major physical abnormalities that occurs with fibromyalgia lies in the muscle itself, where there is a buildup of a protein called "ground substance." Ground substance is normally found in muscle, bone, and connective tissue all over the body and is responsible for making the tissues stronger and less susceptible to tearing. In a normal person, when a muscle is injured, the muscle tissue itself is able to regenerate and, over time, completely heal itself. In a person with fibromyalgia, the muscle is unable to completely heal itself. Instead, an abnormally large amount of ground substance builds up in the injured area which, coupled with the local muscle spasms it creates, produces the muscle "knots" associated with fibromyalgia.

A number of tests may be done to rule out other disorders. Additionally, an examination can reveal whether a person has the characteristic tender areas on the back of the neck, shoulders, sternum, lower back, hips, shins, elbows, or knees. Unlike its cousin lupus, there are no diagnostic laboratory tests for fibromyalgia.

Myofascial Pain Syndrome

Myofascial pain syndrome (MPS), or myofascitis, is characterized by regions of the body that are chronically inflamed, painful, and have multiple trigger points in the muscles. Myofascitis tends to be localized to specific affected areas of the body, such as in the neck and trapezius muscle, whereas fibromyalgia is a condition that simultaneously affects all regions of the body.

Arthritis

The term "arthritis" literally means "joint inflammation." An estimated forty-three million people in the United States suffer from one of the many

---

Fibromyalgia & Myofascial Pain Syndrome Relief!

The DMR Method has proven to be very effective in decreasing the severity and duration of physical pain and disability of fibromyalgia and MPS. The DMR Method effectively decreases muscular stress and irritation by improving mobility, alignment and stability of the effected areas. The treatment often requires a focus on skilled massage and Dynamic Muscle Technique (DMT).

---

different types of arthritis or from other rheumatic conditions; this number is expected to reach sixty million by the year 2020. Only a small percentage of back problems result from arthritis; however, when they do strike, the results can be disabling. Here is an overview of the three most common forms of arthritis that can lead to back and neck pain: osteoarthritis, ankylosing spondylitis, and rheumatoid arthritis.

Osteoarthritis

Osteoarthritis is the most common type of arthritis, affecting an estimated twenty-one million adults in the U.S. It is a chronic disease that leads to the deterioration of joint cartilage (the soft pads of cushioning between the bones in each of your joints) as well as the formation of abnormal bone spurs around the joints. Osteoarthritis primarily affects the weight-bearing joints, such as the knees, hips, and spine. It's common for disc degeneration to also be present when osteoarthritis affects the low back.

Osteoarthritis may first occur without symptoms between thirty and forty years of age, with symptoms generally appearing in middle age. Symptoms typically include joint soreness after periods of activity, and stiffness after periods of rest that goes away quickly when activity resumes. Before the age of fifty-five it occurs equally in both sexes. However, after fifty-five the incidence is higher in women. Systemic symptoms associated with other types of arthritic conditions (e.g., inflammation of the membrane sac surrounding the lungs; surrounding the heart (pericarditis); the heart valves (endocarditis); or the heart muscle (myocarditis)) are generally not associated with osteoarthritis. The effects of osteoarthritis are typically isolated to the joints of the hands and fingers, hips, knees, big toe, and cervical and lumbar spine.

For most people, the cause of osteoarthritis is unknown, but metabolic, genetic, chemical, and mechanical factors all play a role in its development. Osteoarthritis is associated with the aging process and is the most common form of arthritis. The degeneration of the joint may begin as a result of trauma to the joint, occupational overuse, obesity, subluxation, or mal-alignment of the joints (e.g., being bow-legged or knock-kneed).

Rheumatoid Arthritis

Rheumatoid arthritis, commonly referred to as "RA," does not usually affect the spine until the disease is in its later stages; even then it usually just affects the neck. RA is an inflammatory disease of the synovium, or the tissue that encapsulates the joint, resulting in pain, stiffness, swelling, and loss of function of the joints. Rheumatoid arthritis generally occurs in a symmetrical pattern. This means that if one knee or hand is involved, the other one is also. Those who suffer from RA often experience joint pain, fatigue, occasional fever, and a general sense of not feeling well.

Rheumatoid arthritis affects approximately 1 to 2 percent of the total population. The disease can occur at any age, but it most often begins between the ages of twenty-five and fifty-five, and is more common in women. Although the course and the severity of the illness can vary considerably, the onset of the disease is usually gradual, with fatigue, morning stiffness, diffuse muscle aches, loss of appetite, weakness, and, eventually, joint pain. A simple blood test can detect a marker for rheumatoid arthritis called RA factor, the level of which is a fairly good indicator of RA severity.

Like other forms of arthritis, the cause of rheumatoid arthritis is uncertain. However, it is known that RA involves an attack on the body by its own immune cells, which classifies it as an auto-immune condition. Rheumatoid arthritis progresses in three stages. The first stage is the swelling of the synovial lining, causing pain, warmth, stiffness, redness, and swelling around the joint. The second stage is characterized by a thickening of the synovial membrane. In the third stage, the inflamed tissues of the joint release enzymes that break down bone and cartilage, resulting in the progressive destruction of the joint.

Ankylosing Spondylitis

Ankylosing spondylitis (AS) tends to affect people—primarily men—in late adolescence or early adulthood. Ankylosing spondylitis leads to the inflammation and calcification (hardening) of a long, tough ligament that helps to stabilize the spine called the anterior longitudinal ligament. The process of inflammation and calcification causes a slow, progressive loss of mobility in the spine, as well as considerable bouts of back pain. AS may also affect the hips, shoulders, and knees as the tendons and ligaments around the bones and joints become inflamed.

Arthritis Relief!

The vast majority of arthritis cannot be reversed, but there are many things that can be done to help manage symptoms and slow or even stop the progression. If you have an arthritic condition, it's essential that you become proactive in managing your condition. The DMR Method is one of the most effective ways of helping people with arthritic conditions because it safely helps restore maximal mobility, alignment and stability to effected joints-the three key elements to optimal joint health and function.

Ankylosing spondylitis is most common among Native Americans. Often, people with AS are not diagnosed early in the disease process because symptoms are often attributed to more common back problems. The most common early symptom of AS is a dramatic loss of flexibility in the low back. Although most symptoms begin in the lumbar and sacroiliac areas, they may also involve the neck and upper back as well. In a few cases, those with AS experience fever, fatigue, weight loss, anemia, eye inflammation (called iritis), or heart valve problems. Your doctor can do a simple blood test to see if you have the genetic marker (HLA-B27) that is common for a group of conditions called spondyloarthropathies, of which AS is one. Although not all people with the HLA-B27 marker go on to develop AS, it does indicate a predisposition for it.

The cause of ankylosing spondylitis is unknown. For reasons that are not understood, a previous history of urinary tract infections or bowel infections seem to considerably increase the risk of developing AS.

Postural Issues

Postural issues are one of the most common chronic conditions. They can be one of the unfortunate side effects of other spinal conditions, but can also be one of the causes of some other conditions of the spine. For example, people with poor posture become more prone to developing headaches. Understanding the three main postural issues can be helpful in understanding your spinal condition; and the treatment of postural issues can be an essential step in your recovery.

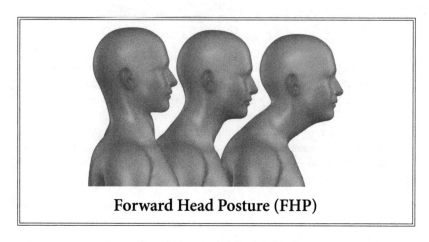

Forward Head Posture (FHP)

Forward head posture (FHP)

Forward head posture (FHP) is the forward positioning of the head and neck relative to the upper back and shoulders. It's also called "scholar's neck," "computer neck," or "reading neck."

FHP can have multiple causes, including sleeping with your head elevated too high, extended computer and cell phone usage, nutrient deficiencies such as low calcium levels, and deconditioned neck, upper back, and shoulder muscles. It is closely associated with conditions called hyperkyphosis and upper crossed syndrome,, in which some muscles become too tight and others become too weak, leading to postural distortion.

Symptoms can include neck, upper back, and shoulder pain; fatigue, tingling, and numbness in the arms; and a burning sensation between the shoulder blades and neck.

Treatment involves correcting any issues with mobility and alignment of the neck and upper back and improving the strength and balance of the supporting muscles. Postural training is also essential.

Hyperkyphosis (Dowagers Hump)

Hyperkyphosis is an abnormal curvature of the thoracic spine leading to an increased bent posture that looks like a hump in the middle of the back. With time it can worsen and cause increasing pain and disability. It is most often caused by poor posture, muscle weakness, spinal degenerative disease, some forms of arthritis, and hereditary factors. It can also be caused by small fractures that occur with osteoporosis, but two-thirds of people with hyperkyphosis do not have spinal fractures. Hyperkyphosis can make a person prone to developing forward head posture (FHP) and upper crossed syndrome.

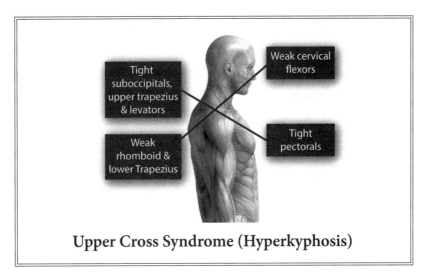

Tight suboccipitals, upper trapezius & levators

Weak cervical flexors

Weak rhomboid & lower Trapezius

Tight pectorals

Upper Cross Syndrome (Hyperkyphosis)

The most prominent symptom of hyperkyphosis is the appearance of a rounded mid back. Initially, the curvature is often mild, but it can progress over time and begin to cause stiffness and pain in the mid back. With further progression, it can cause increasing neck and shoulder pain and can make your lower back prone to injury. In severe cases, it can cause spinal fractures, degenerative fusion of the affected vertebrae, and difficulty with normal breathing.

Treatment includes maximizing mobility and alignment of the spine, stretching and strengthening associated muscles and ligaments, and intensive postural training. A focus on stretching the muscles in the anterior chest and shoulders while strengthening the supportive spine muscles is often essential.

Hyperlordosis

Hyperlordosis occurs when the natural arch in the lower back becomes exaggerated. It is also associated with a condition called lower crossed syndrome because it most often occurs when some supporting muscles become weak and others become tight.

It can also be caused by excessive back extension, trauma, or degenerative disorders in the lumbar spine. It can begin as a mild increase in the lumbar arch; if left untreated it can get progressively worse over time, producing more symptoms and other associated conditions. In addition to causing back pain and stiffness, it can cause or aggravate other conditions such as degenerative disc disease, facet syndrome, disc herniation, stenosis, spondylolisthesis, piriformis syndrome, sciatica, and hip, knee, and foot pain. Treatment focuses on improving mobility and strength to support improved alignment.

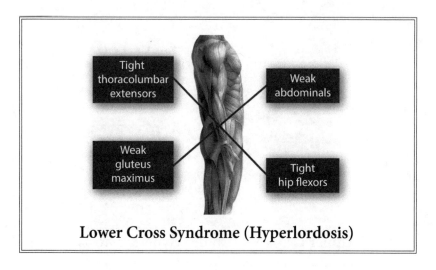

Lower Cross Syndrome (Hyperlordosis)

Inherited (Congenital) Disorders

Scoliosis

Scoliosis is a musculoskeletal disorder that involves an abnormal bending or twisting of the spine. Approximately 80 percent of people with scoliosis have "idiopathic" scoliosis, which means that a particular cause cannot be found. In the remainder of cases, infection, muscle imbalance, or another congenital disorder may be the primary cause. Scoliosis is not necessarily a painful condition if the spine successfully adapts to the abnormal curvature and the curvature is not too severe.

Deciding whether and how much to treat scoliosis depends on several factors, including age, severity, whether the scoliosis is structural (grew that way), or is functional (resulting from an illness or injury), and how much discomfort it causes. Structural scoliosis is only rarely able to be completely corrected. On the other hand, functional scoliosis usually responds well to appropriate treatment. Whether scoliosis is structural or functional, early intervention, proactive management, and proper maintenance care is essential. Because the DMR Method helps maximize mobility, alignment, and stability of the spine, it serves as an effective system of short-term and long-term management of scoliosis.

Spina Bifida

Spina bifida, which literally means "cleft spine," is characterized by the incomplete development of the brain, spinal cord, and/or meninges (the protective covering around the brain and spinal cord). Spina bifida affects fifteen hundred to two thousand babies born in the U.S. each year. There are four types of spina bifida that are categorized by severity:

Spina Bifida Occulta is the mildest and most common form. This type is often discovered incidentally during X-ray evaluation for unrelated spinal conditions and presents as a slight separation of the bone in the back of the lower vertebra or sacrum. This form rarely causes disability or symptoms.

Closed Neural Tube Defects are marked by a malformation of fat tissue, bone, or the membranes surrounding the spinal cord. In some patients there are few or no symptoms; in others the malformation causes partial paralysis with urinary and bowel dysfunction.

Meningocele is marked by the meninges actually protruding from the spinal opening, and may or may not be covered by a layer of skin. Some patients with meningocele have few or no symptoms while others may experience symptoms similar to a closed neural tube defect.

Myelomeningocele is the rarest and most severe form of spina bifida. In this form, the spinal cord is completely exposed through the opening in the spine, resulting in a partial or complete paralysis of the parts of the body below the spinal opening. The paralysis may be so severe that the affected individual is unable to walk and is unable to control bowel and bladder function.

Numerous studies have shown that women who do not consume adequate levels of folic acid are at a greater risk for having children with spina bifida. Because the timing of neural tube development is so early in gestation, by the time women discover that they are pregnant, spina bifida will have already formed if it is going to happen. Consequently, it's important that all women of childbearing age take a good multivitamin with at least 400 mcg of folic acid every day to help reduce the risk of neural tube deficits in their children.

Transitional Vertebrae

Transitional vertebrae are abnormally formed vertebral bones that display the characteristics of two different types of vertebrae. They typically occur at the junction between the cervical and thoracic regions of the spine, or at the junction between the lumbar and sacral regions of the spine. A common form is for the seventh cervical vertebra (C7), which is located adjacent to the first thoracic vertebra (T1), to display some characteristics of a thoracic spinal segment such as having small bumps resembling partially formed ribs attached to the transverse process. Another common type of transitional vertebra occurs between the lowest lumbar vertebra (L5) and the sacrum where L5 becomes partially fused to the sacrum. This is referred to as "sacralization" of the lower lumbar spine. Although most transitional segments do not directly cause pain, they do change the mobility of the affected region and may increase the likelihood of injury or make recovery more difficult.

Nonspinal Conditions

Although most of the research on the DMR Method has been centered around the spine, injuries in other parts of the body can be treated with the DMR Method. Common nonspinal conditions treated with the DMR Method include:

- Shoulder pain and rotator cuff syndrome
- Carpal tunnel syndrome
- Plantar fasciitis
- Sports injuries
- Hip and knee pain/degeneration
- TMJ syndrome

Carpal Tunnel and Plantar Fasciitis— The Spinal Connection

Two common repetitive-use injuries are carpal tunnel syndrome in the wrists and plantar fasciitis in the feet. The carpal tunnel is a small anatomical opening created by the bones of the wrist that allows a bundle of blood vessels, tendons, and nerves to traverse the wrist from the arm to the hand. When the wrists are in a slightly extended position, as they are when typing at a keyboard, the carpal tunnel will collapse slightly, thereby increasing the pressure on the vessels and nerves in the wrist. If this position is held for a long period while the tendons busily move back and forth through the tunnel to move the fingers, the area can become inflamed and swollen. It is this swelling and inflammation that causes the pain associated with carpal tunnel syndrome.

Plantar fasciitis, a type of inflammation that occurs in the feet due to repetitive stress, can be incredibly painful. There are several ligaments in the feet that are responsible for maintaining a healthy arch in bones of the foot; one of these is a thin, sheet-like ligament called the plantar fascia. The plantar fascia is particularly important for keeping the arch of the foot from collapsing while the body is standing, walking, or running. Continuous or repetitive stress of the plantar fascia can result in the tissue becoming damaged and inflamed.

Both of these conditions have a strong connection to overall spinal balance and health. Remember, the nervous system that controls and coordinates all the fine reflexes in the body can be affected by the spine. An imbalance in the nerves that supply the feet and hands can make a person prone to carpal tunnel syndrome and plantar fasciitis. Also, the mobility, alignment, and stability of the spine can cause additional mechanical stress to the arms and legs, making a person prone to these two conditions. Hence, the evaluation and treatment of carpal tunnel syndrome and plantar fasciitis often includes the spine.

Ask Questions

In the next chapter you will learn about the evaluation and treatment approach of the DMR Method. It's essential that you understand your condition and become familiar with every step of the treatment process. The knowledge and understanding you gain will literally help you get healthier. So be sure to ask your providers questions!

DMR Method Case Study - Shoulder Pain & Dysfunction

HISTORY

Christie suffered from severe pain and immobility in her right shoulder. Her symptoms began with repetitive computer and keyboard use at work, and were aggravated every time she reached overhead, reached behind her back, and laid on her right side. She became increasingly disabled at work, was unable to do yard work and gardening without pain, and experienced sleep disturbances.

DIAGNOSIS

DMR Method Evaluation revealed decreased right shoulder range of motion. Muscle strength was decreased and poor shoulder alignment caused the right shoulder blade to displace backwards. Also noted was joint capsule restriction. Positive orthopedic tests indicated tendon damage in the right shoulder.

TREATMENT

Treatment consisted of specific shoulder mobilizations and stretching to improve range of motion and alignment in the shoulder girdle. Interferential electrical stimulation and ice were employed to control inflammation around the shoulder joint. As Christie improved, specific rotator cuff and scapular stabilization strengthening was implemented along with dynamic stabilization exercises and proper posture and body mechanics training.

OUTCOME

The therapist noted restored mobility, alignment and stability in the right shoulder girdle. Christie attained resolution of pain and regained full strength and range of motion in her shoulder. She resumed normal work and home activities without pain. To maintain and stabilize her recovery, she continues to exercise, stretch and use proper posture and body mechanics as instructed by her therapist. Her 16-month follow-up revealed that she was pain-free and fully functional.

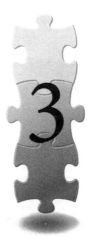

The DMR Method

The DMR Method, which is a specialized system to Diagnose, Manage, and Rehabilitate neck and back pain, is the culmination of more than twenty-five years of clinical experience in treating thousands of patients suffering from back and neck pain. That period included years of clinical research that analyzed changes in functional index scores (which track a person's ability to engage in normal physical activities) and both pre-treatment and post-treatment MRI evaluations. The DMR Method, a tightly structured evaluation and treatment protocol, has an extraordinary success rate in decreasing both short-term and long-term pain and disability. While many of the individual techniques that comprise the DMR Method are known to most healthcare providers, four particular aspects differentiate the process from other spine therapy programs:

- The DMR Method evaluation and treatment protocol leverages the expertise of three different types of healthcare providers—physical therapists, chiropractors, and medical doctors—who have been trained to work together on behalf of, and in cooperation with, the patient.

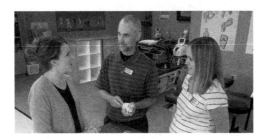

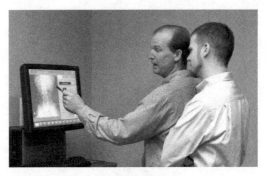

- The DMR Method evaluation is a customized, detailed process of identifying the root cause of each individual patient's condition and all the factors that may influence recovery.

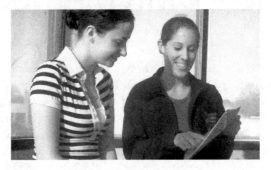

- The DMR Method includes a unique progression of joint manipulation (Integrated Progressive Manipulation), soft-tissue massage (Dynamic Muscle Technique), and traction (DMR Method Progressive Traction) provided by a collaborative team of healthcare providers.

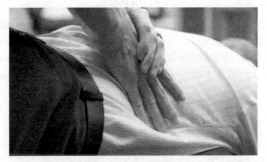

- Treatment involves a comprehensive and specific path of clinical care and self-care that provides the right modality in the right order to produce rapid, predictable, and positive results.

It's Easier Than You Think!

The DMR Method is a detailed process of evaluation and treatment that at first may sound a bit overwhelming. But trust me on this: it's easier than you may think and the results are definitely worth the effort! Patients who have struggled with pain and disability for years and have been through an endless cycle of failed tests and treatments often say to me after beginning care, "I can't believe it was so easy to feel good again."

Why is getting healthy again so easy? Three reasons: First, most of the DMR Method evaluation and treatment process is organized and performed by your DMR Method treatment team. Second, your DMR Method providers will educate and guide you through the DMR Method process with great care, compassion, and empathy. Third, when the time comes for you to begin a self-care program, you'll have a clear understanding of what you need to do and why you need to do it.

Understanding the DMR Method evaluation and treatment process, starts with understanding the importance of the treatment sequence.

Treatment Sequence

To illustrate why the treatment sequence is so crucial, think of your recovery as similar to the process of building a house. You begin by establishing a foundation, building the frame, and then installing such things as siding, roofing, plumbing, and flooring. Those steps need to be performed in the right order; laying the flooring before pouring the foundation will lead to a sub-optimal outcome!

The same dynamic applies to care of the body. Trying to perform certain exercises or stretches before the body is ready can reduce, eliminate, or even sabotage the expected benefits of those activities. Rehabilitative exercise-based programs that rely on extensive and often machine-assisted exercises may provide initial relief, but can ultimately backfire if the underlying cause of the condition was not corrected first. Indeed, introducing certain stretches or exercises too quickly can trigger a relapse into pain and disability.

Case in point: a long-distance runner who came in for evaluation of his hip and lower back pain had previously seen a sports medicine doctor who prescribed an aggressive strengthening program. Initially it seemed to work and he was able to resume running; soon, however, his back and hip pain returned in full force and his knee began hurting as well. Although the strengthening program had been well designed by a competent physical therapist, it was ultimately counterproductive. A DMR Method evaluation

---

BIG IDEA! *Mobility, Alignment, and Stability*

All symptomatic musculoskeletal conditions of the spine, whether acute or chronic, are the result of altered mobility, alignment, and stability of the affected muscles, ligaments, joints, or disc tissues. Effective treatment of all conditions of the spine focuses on the maximal restoration of Mobility, Alignment, and Stability (MAS)—not just one of them, but all of them. A key point is that these have to be restored in the exact order of Mobility first, Alignment second, and Stability third. This produces the best results and doing MAS out of order is often the reason why a person doesn't enjoy full recovery.

---

revealed that his left leg was three-quarters of an inch shorter than his right. Consequently, his running regimen threw his back and pelvis out of alignment and caused him to bear excessive weight on his left leg, which led to hip and knee pain. After instructing him to stop exercising, we provided him with a lift to correct his leg length discrepancy, restored mobility and alignment to his spine and pelvis through chiropractic treatment and physical therapy, and only then had him resume his strengthening program. That was more than a decade ago and he is still running marathons to this day.

Paying Attention to Detail

Back in the 1980s, Ford Motor Company bought an interest in the Japanese automobile company, Mazda. In fact, some of the cars and trucks Ford sold during this time were made by Mazda but were sold under the Ford name. Shortly after the two companies began working together, the management at Ford noticed that the transmissions manufactured in their Ford plant had seven times the rate of breakdown than those made in the Mazda plant. Because of their partnership, Ford happened to have some of the Mazda transmissions on hand and decided to take a closer look.

The officials at Ford initially thought that Mazda had changed the design in some way and that these changes were responsible for the dramatic increase in durability. However, once they pulled open the transmission and the inspectors measured everything, they discovered that Mazda had followed the Ford blueprints exactly. So exact, in fact, that every component in each transmission was exactly the same size.

The engineers at first thought there was something wrong with their testing equipment, but they soon discovered that the Mazda transmissions were indeed built to extraordinarily tight tolerances. The blueprints provided to Mazda allowed a tolerance of plus or minus a few percentage for each part, which meant that there was an allowable deviation in the specifications of each part. While all of the American-made transmission parts were within these allowable tolerances, the Japanese-made gears were all exactly on the desired value with only a negligible amount of variation. The executives at Ford were shocked by the difference that this tiny detail made.

What they discovered is a general principle of complex systems: details matter. They matter because the additive effect of many small defects can lead to the entire system failing. This principle not only applies to transmissions, rockets, and computers, it also applies to biological systems like the human body. While not eating the best foods, not getting as much exercise as you should, not having the best posture, or experiencing daily stress may not lead to a significant breakdown of the body when experienced individually, they can dramatically increase your likelihood of physical breakdown when combined with each other.

One of the things you will notice as you go through the DMR Method is how structured and detailed the process is. The components of the DMR acronym: *Diagnose, Manage and Rehabilitate*, represent the key steps in developing the correct progression of coordinated care. Favorable outcomes will only be achieved if every aspect of the biological system that is your body is fully and carefully addressed. Like in the Ford-Mazda transmission experience, it is the cumulative effect of making sure that all of your parts are operating as they should that makes your body resilient, strong, and fully functional.

In this chapter, you will be introduced to the DMR Method evaluation and treatment protocol. You'll learn why a thorough history and examination are integral to the development of the most effective treatment program, what to expect during your recovery, and why every component of the process is so critical to recovery.

The DMR Method of Evaluation

Regardless of your final diagnosis, our goal is to identify how it has affected the mobility, alignment, and stability of your spine, and to develop a treatment plan that restores optimal mobility, alignment, and stability. If we are successful, you will get rapid relief of your symptoms and learn how to keep feeling great from that moment forward. This is true even for complicated cases that have failed to improve with other forms of treatment.

Health History

Dr. William Osler, a famous physician from the late 19th century, often advised new classes of medical students to "listen to your patients, for they are telling you the diagnosis." In other words, by engaging in a conversation with a patient about their condition, the healthcare provider can learn a tremendous amount about what may be contributing to the issues at hand. Although this seems obvious to us today, at that time actually listening to what the patient had to say was a novel idea. Up to that point, doctors just assumed that they could perform a couple of tests, listen to the patient's lungs, hit their knee with a reflex hammer, and deduce the problem. No wonder so many treatments failed back then!

The surest way to accurately understand the source of your discomfort is to initiate a conversation with you. As part of this process, you may be asked about many things, such as:

- *Onset.* When and how did this issue start? Did it come on suddenly or slowly? What were you doing when the pain started? Have you had this before? Certain conditions tend to have an identifiable onset. For example, if you were shovelling dirt in your garden and felt a "snap" in your low back, this gives your healthcare provider important insight into your condition.

- *Quality and grade of pain.* Is your pain sharp or a dull ache? Is the degree of pain an annoyance, or are you completely debilitated? This helps us understand if there is a nerve being impinged, whether there is a lot of inflammation, or whether some of your internal organs are being affected.

- *What makes the pain worse or better?* Identifying what makes your pain worse or better provides your healthcare provider with valuable information about the source of the pain. For example, if you have a ruptured disc in your low back that is pressing on a nerve, standing in certain positions will often provide some relief from pain. However, if the source of pain is purely from inflammation, different postures may accentuate the pain rather than providing relief.

- *Does the pain radiate?* There are certain conditions in which pain may be experienced in one part of the body, but the actual cause of the problem is somewhere else. For example, the symptoms of a heart attack may be experienced as pain in the left arm; a gallbladder attack is often experienced as pain in the right shoulder; and shooting pain down the back of the leg may be due to a muscle spasm in the buttock.

- *Timing*—when does it hurt? Is your pain better in the morning but worsens throughout the day, or just the opposite? Are you pain free on a particular day of the week? The timing of your pain can provide valuable information about external stressors that may be contributing to your pain. It is not uncommon for people with a worn-out mattress to have low-back pain in the morning which steadily improves as the day wears on. Alternatively, people with inflammatory conditions may wake up feeling great, only to have their pain return as they participate in daily activities.

- *Lifestyle habits.* Most people are aware that habits such as smoking, lack of exercise, poor diet, watching too much TV, or lack of sleep are bad for the body. However, most do not understand how harmful some of these activities can be. Smoking, for example, causes constriction of the tiny blood vessels that help keep the spinal discs in the low back fully hydrated and healthy. Smokers will experience more low-back pain than non-smokers simply because of the impact that smoking has on blood circulation. Although many people do not want to admit to their doctor that they smoke, eat fast food, consume several soft drinks per day, and don't exercise, this is valuable information that your health-care professional needs to know to fully understand your condition.

- *Supplements and medications.* Anything you put in your body is going to influence your physical health. From the quantity of water you drink to the vitamins you take to the chemicals absorbed during a round of chemotherapy, every substance that is internalized will impact how your body works. Because medications and supplements tend to be compounds that have a stronger impact on your health, gram for gram, compared to a substance like water, it's important to have an accurate picture of what external chemicals may be either helping or exacerbating your condition.

- *Past medical or treatment history.* A complete picture of your past health issues and treatments is particularly valuable in identifying potential contributing factors to your current condition, limitations to evaluation and treatment, and possible roadblocks to recovery. Back surgery, for example, may limit the type of diagnostic imaging that can be performed or what type of therapy can be employed.

- *Pain and disability indexes.* These forms are usually completed at the beginning of treatment and then periodically updated throughout treatment. They are intended to evaluate how your current condition is impacting your life. Are you able to take care of yourself? How much pain are you experiencing in different situations? This information helps your doctor identify particular areas of disability and to create and revise treatment plans that restore functionality as quickly as possible. Standardized indexes are also valuable in quantifying the rate and degree of recovery.

The process of providing so much information may seem tedious. However, building an accurate diagnosis and appropriate plan of treatment and rehabilitation depends on good information—and a lot of it. The human body is a complex system and the language it speaks to give us feedback is pain. It takes a lot of information to figure out what the body is trying to say.

A doctor friend of mine once told me about one of the first patients he saw after graduating from chiropractic school. The patient was a healthy, athletic young woman who was around seventeen years old. She had awakened with back pain the morning after a soccer match in which she had slipped on the wet grass and fallen on her hip at what she described as a "weird angle."

She stated that she hadn't had any back pain prior to the fall, so he assumed it was a pretty simple case. A cursory examination showed that she had a lot of muscle spasm in her low back and the pain felt "about the same" no matter what position she was in. Aside from describing her pain as "deep" and "dull," everything pointed to a muscle injury in her low back, so that's what he started treating her for.

A week later, the young woman had not improved and, in fact, had stopped coming in to see him. When she finally returned with her mother three weeks later, he learned that the source of the young woman's pain was actually a kidney infection and not a low-back injury. He now is much more thorough with every patient.

Patty's Story

My neck was a wreck due to three bulging discs. I couldn't turn my head from side to side or lift my head off of a pillow without using my hand to do so. My neck was tight, painful and debilitating. I was told repeatedly by friends and family that I would have to have surgery. I didn't want to go that route and was encouraged to hear there was an alternative to surgery called the DMR Method. The expertise and help I received from the physical therapists, chiropractors, and massage therapists brought healing and restoration.   You are all amazing! Thank you so much!

- Patty N.
Hopkins, MN

The moral of this true story is that sometimes symptoms may appear to be caused by one thing, but they may actually be indicative of something else. There are times when it may seem obvious that a particular activity or event caused the problem you are currently experiencing. However, allow me to emphasize that association does not equal causation. Although the timing of the young woman's back pain was associated with an awkward fall the previous evening, it does not mean that her fall was the cause of her pain. I keep this story in mind when I encourage my patients to be honest and thorough when providing information about their health history.

Exam

After completing your health history, it's important to undergo a physical examination. A thorough history will have provided enough information for your doctor to have a pretty good idea about what's going on and where your particular problems may reside. However, it's still necessary to gather more information to either confirm or disconfirm this hypothesis and to look for signs that may indicate other problems. A physical exam is comprised of several steps. Let's take a brief look at each of them.

- *The Basics.* Most healthcare clinics will perform a series of simple tests to determine your general state of health (e.g., taking your pulse, temperature, blood pressure, height, weight, and body fat percentage). These may not seem immediately relevant to someone who just injured their back shovelling snow, but any abnormality in these tests can indicate any larger underlying problems that may impede your recovery. For example, hypothyroid may be indicated by a low body temperature, weight gain, and sensitivity to cold. That particular condition can also reduce your ability to heal.

- *Posture.* Believe it or not, the simple act of carefully evaluating your posture can provide considerable information about what's going on at a functional level. It's not uncommon for people in pain to lean to one side or the other in an effort to be more comfortable or to carry their head forward. Other things to look for include one shoulder being higher than the other, or spinal irregularities such as scoliosis. Each distortion of posture has both causes and consequences.

- *Range of motion.* Range of motion refers to your ability to move. How far can you turn your head or bend at the waist? Is it the same from side to side? One of the markers used to determine the severity of any condition is the degree to which it affects your ability to move normally. People with low-back pain, for example, often find it painful to bend at the waist in one direction, but not the other. As your recovery progresses, your range of motion should improve. In fact, changes in range of motion is one of the factors we use to track your progress.

- *Neurological tests.* You've probably experienced a doctor hitting you on the knee with a little rubber hammer and watching your leg jump a little. Your leg jumped because the tiny nerve endings inside the tendon in your knee are stimulated whenever the tendon is stretched, which occurs when your knee is struck by a rubber hammer. This stretch, in turn, causes the attached muscles to contract. At least, that's what's supposed to happen. There are some conditions, however, in which this reflex is either diminished—as can be the case when a nerve is impinged—or accentuated, which can indicate a central nervous system problem. Testing the sensation in specific areas on your skin (called dermatomes) and testing the strength of certain muscles can also assist in identifying the specific nerves that are causing or contributing to your condition.

- *Orthopedic tests.* These tests involve putting your body into several different positions to help clarify the source of your condition. During this part of the exam you may be asked to take several steps on your heels or toes, or tuck your chin to your chest while the doctor lifts up your arm and checks your pulse. The doctor may also turn your upper body and have you lean back while putting pressure on your spine. Each of these actions is intended to provide information about what's going on with your muscles, bones, nerves, and blood vessels. If a particular test elicits pain or is difficult to do, it gives your doctor insight into where the source of your problems resides.

- *Palpation.* Palpation, which means "feeling with the hands," is an invaluable component of the DMR Method evaluation. Performed by both the evaluating chiropractor and physical therapist, it provides essential information about the structure of your spine. Palpation in this context has three goals:

  1) Evaluate the supportive muscles for their tenderness, tone, and symmetry.

  2) Test and analyze the mobility of each segment of the spine, which is done by applying a light stress to each segment of the spine while the patient relaxes.

  3) Evaluate the alignment and balance of the entire spine and each individual segment.

Big Idea! The Power of Palpation

Remember, one of the keys to the success of the DMR Method is the treatment of abnormal mobility, alignment and stability of the spine. Skilled hands-on palpation by a team of physical therapists and chiropractors is the most powerful tool in identifying deficient mobility, alignment and stability. Palpation is such a powerful tool that it is performed each and every visit during the DMR Method as a means of tracking progress.

- *Diagnostic testing.* Diagnostic testing is a general term that refers to any test that requires analytical equipment to complete. In this category are tests such as X-rays, magnetic resonance imaging (MRI), blood tests, urinalysis, electromyograms, and the like. X-rays and MRIs are the most common diagnostic tests performed during the DMR Method evaluation. X-rays are useful for seeing the relationship between the bones in the body, as well as for identifying bone fractures and other abnormalities, which can be enormously helpful in visualizing mechanical problems in the spine and joints. One concern for some patients is the exposure to radiation that X-rays produce. However, the level of radiation used in current X-ray machines is negligible. In fact, you are exposed to more radiation during most airplane flights due to being higher up in the atmosphere than from a typical series of X-rays. MRIs do not use radiation at all; instead, they leverage strong magnetic fields to produce images. The advantage of MRIs is the added ability to examine muscle, spinal discs, and connective tissue. The downside is the cost: MRIs are much more expensive than X-rays.

DMR Method Innovation: Proprioceptometry™

The DMR Method research team has developed, and is currently testing a diagnostic test that measures something called "Proprioception." Proprioception is basically your bodies ability to automatically balance and coordinate posture and movement. This is important to the DMR Method because when joints in your body aren't moving or aligned properly, proprioception declines. So, if proprioception can be measured, it becomes a tool to not only help diagnose, but a tool to help measure objective improvement as you recover!

DMR Diagnosis and Report of Findings

Once all of the information is gathered from your history, examination, and any additional diagnostics, your doctor will be equipped to make a fairly accurate determination about the severity, cause, and course of treatment for your particular situation. Assuming that the evaluation is done properly, your healthcare provider will be able to design a treatment plan that will provide optimal relief in the shortest amount of time. The first step is for your doctor to do a report of findings in which they spend some time explaining their findings and provide you with a detailed plan of care. During the report of findings your doctor will answer these four basic questions:

- Can you help me?

- How are you going to help me?

- What do I have to do as part of my recovery?

- How long it will likely take me to get well?

Typically, the report of findings will be presented to you on a follow-up visit to allow your doctor sufficient time to analyze the test results and to determine the most effective course of treatment.

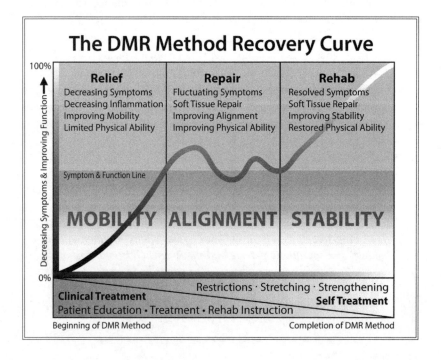

The DMR Method Recovery Curve

100%

Decreasing Symptoms & Improving Function ↑

Relief	Repair	Rehab
Decreasing Symptoms	Fluctuating Symptoms	Resolved Symptoms
Decreasing Inflammation	Soft Tissue Repair	Soft Tissue Repair
Improving Mobility	Improving Alignment	Improving Stability
Limited Physical Ability	Improving Physical Ability	Restored Physical Ability

Symptom & Function Line

MOBILITY | ALIGNMENT | STABILITY

0%

Restrictions · Stretching · Strengthening

Clinical Treatment   **Self Treatment**
Patient Education • Treatment • Rehab Instruction

Beginning of DMR Method   Completion of DMR Method

The DMR Method Recovery Curve

Before delving into the details of the DMR Method treatment program, I'd like to take a moment to explain how the body recovers from injury. Any time your body suffers an injury, whether from some type of trauma such as a car accident, a repetitive-use injury such as carpal tunnel syndrome, or a degenerative disorder such as a bulged lumbar disc, there are three primary areas of function affected: mobility, alignment, and stability. The primary goal of the DMR Method is to restore normal mobility, alignment, and stability to the body—in that order.

If proper treatment is provided, recovery will follow a predictable path of decreasing symptoms and improved function. The recovery progresses through three phases: relief, repair, and rehabilitation (rehab). The DMR Method Recovery Curve graphic, which was developed based on the clinical observation of thousands of patients, is used as a patient education tool. It's also used clinically to keep patients and their providers coordinated and on track. Let's take a look at the three individual phases of recovery.

Relief

In this first phase of care, the goal is to provide some measure of relief from your pain, decrease inflammation, and start the process of restoring normal mobility to the injured areas of your body. During this phase, your DMR Method provider will give you guidance on how to safely perform certain physical activities. He or she may also set limits on some of those activities to ensure that you won't aggravate your condition. This may be necessary for a couple of reasons. First, when injured, muscles, ligaments, and tendons are weakened and more susceptible to additional injury. In this weakened state, even things as simple as lifting groceries out of the car, vacuuming the floor, doing laundry, or even sitting for prolonged periods can cause further damage. It is therefore often necessary to either limit or modify your day-to-day activities to avoid placing additional stress on injured area of your body.

Second, injured tissues will become inflamed. Inflammation is the enemy of swift and proper healing. While inflammation is a natural process, it is an evolutionary carryover from the days when hygiene and access to clean anything was not what it is today. People were hunter-gatherers for the vast majority of human history, and during most of human history the number one killer by far was infection. In order to survive, the human body needed to develop a way to constantly fight bacteria and viruses. One of the ways the

---

BIG IDEA! Pain-Free is not Problem-Free

Most people are under the assumption that if they don't feel any pain that there is nothing wrong with them – that they are healthy. Unfortunately, pain is a very poor indicator of health. In fact, pain and other symptoms frequently only appear after a disease or other condition has become advanced. For example, consider a cavity in your tooth. Does it hurt when it first develops or after it has become serious? How about heart disease, diabetes or cancer? Many times there are little or no symptoms in the early stages of these diseases. Regardless of whether you are talking about cancer, heart disease, diabetes, stress or problems with the spine, pain is usually the last thing to appear. When you begin the DMR Method, pain is many times the first symptom to disappear, even though much of the underlying condition remains.

---

body does this is through inflammation. The problem is that inflammation, while helpful in killing off invading microbes, is not particularly helpful in making sure that tissues heal properly. It's important during this initial phase of treatment that any inflammation in the injured areas is reduced. As will be discussed later, this is done through a variety of techniques such as the use of ice, cold-laser therapy, anti-inflammatory supplements, and protecting the area from re-injury.

Repair

The second phase of recovery is the repair phase. During this phase, your pain will have improved significantly although you may still have periods of flare-up, your soft tissues are going through stages of repair, your posture and

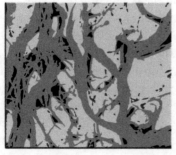
Damaged Ligament

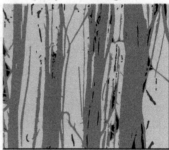
Properly Healed Ligament

alignment should be improving, and you will find it easier to do the things you like to do. Unfortunately, it is also a time when many people decide that they have fully recovered and discontinue their treatment.

Why is this a problem? The graphic shown on the previous page shows a microscopic view of a ligament that has been injured. On the left, you can see how the fibers look like a chaotic mess; this is how damaged tissue repairs itself when it isn't managed properly and scar tissue forms. On the right side is the result of a damaged ligament that has been treated properly; notice that the fibers are straight and organized.

Ligaments are similar to rope. They tie the joints of the body together. If the picture shown on the previous page was showing ropes, which one would look stronger: the pile of frayed scraps or the straight, organized, and unfrayed ones? Your decision to either continue or discontinue treatment during this phase will determine which picture will resemble your tissues. As you begin to feel better, it's important not to be lulled into a false sense of recovery and resume physical activity for which your body is not yet ready.

Rehab

The third phase of the DMR Method is the rehab phase. During this phase, your symptoms will likely be completely resolved, you can engage in your normal daily activities, and your body will have mostly healed from your injury. However, there is still work to be done to reduce your risk of re-injury. Some areas of recovery, such as soft-tissue strength and neurological coordination, require a longer-term approach. During this phase, you will be engaging in more physically intense activities to help promote stability and proper coordination.

BIG IDEA! The 11-18 Month Rule

Even though symptoms are typically resolved at the conclusion of the DMR Method treatment program, patients must continue with appropriate restrictions and be consistent with self-care for a minimum of 11-18 months. Ligaments, one of the main stabilizers of the joints in your body, take 11-18 months to heal. So, if you do too much too soon or stop doing the prescribed self-care, your condition could return.

DMR Method® Treatment Progression

Phase	Relief Phase I	Repair Phase II	Rehab Phase III
Schedule	Visit 1-12 (3x/week)	Visit 13-19 (2x/week)	Visit 20-24 (1x/week)
Clinical Care	**Phase I Clinical Care** + Patient education, lifestyle and body mechanics training + Pain/Inflammation management + Integrated Progressive Mobilization (IPM) level 1 + Dynamic Muscle Technique (DMT)* + Decompression traction* + Cold Laser and EMS Therapy* + Phase I integrated stretching and flexibility techniques	**Phase II Clinical Care** + DMR Method progress evaluation + Integrated care plan update + Integrated Progressive Mobilization (IPM) level 2/3 + Progressed lifestyle and body mechanics training + Advanced stretch instruction + Static exercise instruction and implementation	**Phase III Clinical Care** + DMR Method progress evaluation 2 + Integrated care plan update 2 + Integrated Progressive Mobilization (IPM) level 3 + Dynamic exercise instruction and implementation + Personalized self care program instruction + Graduation from DMR Method
Self Care	**Phase I Self Care** + Home care and restrictions + Proper body mechanics * + Supportive nutrition * + Phase I stretching	**Phase II Self Care** + Updated restrictions + Phase II stretching + Static exercises	**Phase III Self Care** + Return to normal activities + Dynamic and proprioceptive exercises
Goal	MOBILITY	ALIGNMENT	STABILITY

* Continues through entire DMR Method treatment progression

DMR Method Treatment Progression

Each phase of your recovery—relief, repair, and rehab—employs a series of therapies to help restore mobility, alignment, and stability, which is the central goal of the DMR Method. The success of the DMR Method lies in the use of therapies performed in a specific order and at the right frequency and combination over an appropriate time period. The graphic above highlights the more common therapies and self-care activities during each phase of treatment. Let's explore each of these therapies so you understand how they can help you recover.

Lifestyle & Self-Care Techniques

Here are brief overviews of some lifestyle and self-care techniques used in the DMR Method. You can learn more about each of these techniques later in the book or from your care providers. In chapter 4, "Your DMR Method Program," you'll find information boxes that you and your DMR Method provider can use to help you organize and understand all of the elements of your individual treatment and recovery program.

Restrictions and Limitations

Reducing the stress on an injured body part is an important step in the overall recovery process. Restricting the use of affected areas of the body not only reduces the risk of re-injury, it allows you to focus on healing those parts of the body. A complete guide to appropriate restrictions and limitations is included in chapter 5.

Orthopedic Braces and Supports

At times, an injury may require the use of an orthopedic brace, support, or other adaptive tool to assist in recovery. These tools will help create the perfect environment for your body to focus on healing.

Lifestyle Training

Have you ever stopped to think how much your daily activities impact your body? Most people don't realize how sitting for long periods of time, sleeping on their stomach, or bending and twisting while lifting can significantly increase their chance of injury and impede their recovery should injury

Dave's Story

From the moment I was greeted by the friendly front desk staff until I had my final physical therapy session, I knew I had found the right place to help me with my three bulging discs. For the past nine months I wasn't able to fully enjoy snow skiing, barefoot water skiing, and biking. After an initial consultation and X-ray, I was presented with a DMR Method treatment plan that included physical therapy and chiropractic adjustments.

The physical therapy consisted of cold laser treatment to help encourage muscle and tissue repair, massage, stretching, strength exercises to improve my core, and lastly, traction. After about six weeks of treatment, my back feels great and I feel ten years younger. I've incorporated the exercises and stretching into my weekly workouts to help maintain a healthy back and core.

- Dave C.
Minneapolis, MN

occur. Learning better ways to position and move your body throughout the day can help facilitate your recovery and reduce the chances of re-injury. A complete guide to proper body mechanics and lifestyle techniques are included in chapter 5. Your DMR Method providers will select the techniques that are essential to your recovery.

Stretching

The DMR Method includes a unique system of progressive stretching and flexibility techniques that were designed to help patients stretch safely and effectively through all three phases of the DMR Method. Following an injury, therapeutic stretching can prevent scar tissue from forming. During and after recovery, maintaining a regular stretching program helps keep tissues flexible, increases mobility, and protects you from new injuries.

Exercise

Three types of exercise are part of the DMR Method: strength, aerobic, and proprioceptive. Strength exercises are especially useful for improving posture, muscle balance, and, of course, strength. Aerobic exercise helps develop endurance. Low-intensity, long-duration aerobic exercises include walking, climbing stairs, and bicycling.

Proprioceptive exercises help your body improve its natural ability to balance itself. Benefits include improved alignment, posture, coordination, and balance. The DMR Method incorporates both strength and aerobic forms of proprioceptive exercises.

Beginning the strengthening portion of treatment too soon, or doing the wrong combination of exercises, are two of the most common roadblocks to recovery. In designing the appropriate DMR Method protocol for your condition, your healthcare providers will develop a specific, step-by-step program that includes all three types of exercise.

Nutritional Therapy

Nutrition is an often-overlooked aspect of recovery. The right nutrients provide the building blocks that the body needs to repair itself following an injury. Just like having the right building materials to repair your home following storm damage, your body needs the correct materials to maximize the degree and rate of recovery.

During recovery from any injury, the body has an increased demand for certain vitamins and minerals. By supplementing a healthy diet with these nutrients, you're providing your body with the support it needs to heal properly. Micro-minerals are especially important because they support wound healing, but little trace of them is found in the typical American diet. Zinc, one of the more difficult minerals to obtain dietarily, is utilized by over two hundred enzymes involved in metabolism, DNA repair, and tissue construction. When you're injured, your body kicks your metabolism into high gear in order to repair itself as quickly as possible; if adequate supplies of zinc are not present, your body won't be able to heal correctly.

As part of your DMR Method program, you'll be given dietary guidelines to aid in your recovery, including a list of foods that enhance recovery and foods to avoid. If additional supplementation is necessary based upon your individual needs, your doctor or physical therapist will discuss how each particular supplement will help you. As with all other parts of your DMR Method recovery program, there is a specific purpose behind every recommendation and treatment.

Relief and Repair Packs

Relief and Repair Packs are a GMP-certified nutritional supplement that were developed and formulated by the DMR Method research team. (Good manufacturing practices (GMP) are the practices required to conform to guidelines recommended by agencies that control authorization and licensing for manufacture and sale of food, drug products, and active pharmaceutical products.) In addition to a multivitamin and micronutrients formulation that was specifically designed to support soft-tissue healing and repair, the packs include:

Glucosamine and Chondroitin

Glucosamine and chondroitin are precursors for a compound called glycosaminoglycan, a major component of joint cartilage. When joints become injured, the inflammation that results causes a degradation of the cartilage. Because cartilage is so critical for healthy joint motion, any damage can lead to a loss of joint function. By providing the building blocks for joint cartilage, glucosamine and chondroitin helps the joint cartilage heal.

MSM (Methylsulfonylmethane)

MSM is a natural source of sulfur for the body, which can be helpful in recovering from a musculoskeletal injury. Sulfur is normally found in onions, garlic, cruciferous vegetables, and high-protein foods such as eggs, nuts, seeds, and milk. Sulfur is a "strengthening agent" used by the body during the production of bone, muscle, and connective tissue. It works by forming links between strands of protein called "disulfide bonds." These bonds essentially work by taking strands of protein strings and tying them together into a net, thereby dramatically increasing the overall strength and resilience of your tissues.

Beyond its role in maintaining tissue health and strength, MSM is often used as a therapy for a variety of conditions, including inflammation, arthritis, and the stimulation of wound healing. Although there is no recommended dietary allowance (RDA) established for dietary sulfur, several nutritional researchers have stated that the typical American may be getting inadequate levels of organic sulfur in their diet. Because MSM is a safe compound and provides a variety of health benefits, it's include in our Relief and Repair Packs.

Trypsin and Chymotrypsin

Trypsin and chymotripsin are powerful proteolytic enzymes, which means they work to break down proteins. While these enzymes perform several important digestive and signalling functions in the body, they also have a powerful anti-inflammatory effect following an injury.

Calcium and Magnesium

Calcium, which plays a key role in the strength and structural integrity of

---

Fish and Water Go Together!

Your DMR Method provider will discuss with you the importance of drinking a lot of clean water during your recovery. Keeping your body hydrated is essential and it will help optimize all the physiological processes that are taking place during your recovery. Your provider may also talk to you about the benefits of fish oil. Fish Oil contains omega-3 fatty acids and it's one of the most popular supplements because of it's benefits regarding cardiovascular health. But research on omega-3 fatty acids suggests that they also decrease the inflammation associated with injury and arthritis, and they are helpful in protecting the nervous system from stress-related injury.

DMR Method™ Case Study

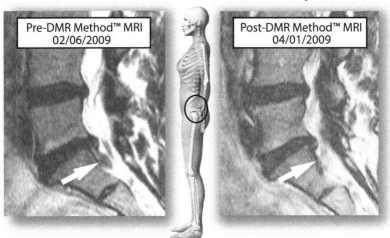

Pre-DMR Method™ MRI
02/06/2009

Post-DMR Method™ MRI
04/01/2009

Moderate Disc Herniation Lumbar Spine

Laura, who has a history of rheumatoid arthritis, was in an exercise class when she felt her back give out. The pain worsened over the next few hours and began causing numbness and weakness in her left leg. She couldn't bear weight on her left leg and couldn't sit, stand or walk without severe lower back and leg pain.

DIAGNOSIS

An MRI scan revealed a moderate left-sided L5-S1 disc herniation with nerve root compression. DMR Method Evaluation revealed severe immobility and misalignment of the lower lumbar spine and pelvis, plus muscle spasm, swelling, and remodeling/constriction of the muscles and ligaments in the lower lumbar spine and pelvis.

TREATMENT

Acute Lumbar DMR Protocol. Laura was also referred for a lumbar epidural injection to decrease acute pain and inflammation.

OUTCOME

Laura attained complete resolution of back and leg symptoms and returned to aggressive fitness activities. A follow-up MRI eight weeks after her initial MRI revealed complete reabsorption of the disc herniation. Her five-year follow-up revealed continued symptom resolution. Her arthritis-related back pain has been managed with stretching and periodic care. She maintains a very active lifestyle and manages her rheumatoid arthritis well.

bone, is also used in nerve transmission and muscle contraction. Magnesium is an essential component in many enzymatic reactions and is also an important modulator in wound healing. Deficiencies in magnesium can interfere with wound healing and tissue repair. Calcium and magnesium together can support healthy muscle contraction and decrease muscle spasm.

Clinical Care Techniques

While many of the lifestyle and self-care techniques described in this book are intended to be continued for a lifetime, clinical care techniques are the essential treatment components performed by DMR Method practitioners over the initial stages of treatment. This structured, coordinated progression of clinical care is designed to decrease symptoms; improve mobility, alignment, and stability; and teach patients how to maintain their recovery beyond the clinical care phase. Separately, each of these elements has its own benefits, but together—in the right combination and the right order—they can produce amazing results. Many of these clinical techniques are standard treatments in the healthcare industry, but have been refined to fit into a specific progression and combination. These core clinical care techniques include:

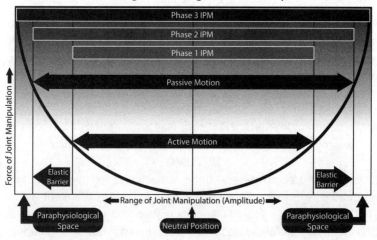

DMR Method chiropractors developed this physiological model of joint motion and manipulation as the basis of Integrated Progressive Manipulation.

Integrated Progressive Manipulation (IPM)

Integrated Progressive Manipulation is a safe, highly effective progression of joint mobilization developed by the chiropractors involved with DMR Method development and research. IPM progresses through three phases of manipulation in synchronization with other elements of DMR Method protocols.

IPM safely improves joint mobility and alignment with minimal stress to the joints and supportive soft tissue. IPM is a form of chiropractic adjustment, the goal of which is to reduce subluxations.

Subluxation refers to any alteration in mobility or alignment of a joint that affects the ability of the joint to function normally. A subluxation can also cause an imbalance in the local or peripheral nervous system.

The local nervous system (aka proprioception) refers to the part of the nervous system that senses movement, pressure, and tension in the affected joints, associated muscles, ligaments, and other supportive soft tissues. It provides vital information to help your brain coordinate and control movement, balance, and posture. Dysfunction in the local nervous system causes imbalance, loss of coordination, and overstressing of the affected joints, associated muscles, ligaments, and other supportive soft tissues.

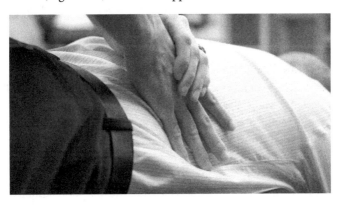

The peripheral nervous system refers to the nerves that are in close proximity to the affected joints but don't have a direct connection with them. If these peripheral nerves are affected by altered mobility or alignment, the patient may experience pain and other adverse symptoms and nerve dysfunction.

Integrated Progressive Manipulations are applied by hand to gently reduce subluxations to the affected joints. The three phases of manipulation are graduated to gently progress further and further into the full range of motion of joints as the flexibility of the muscles, ligaments, and other supportive soft

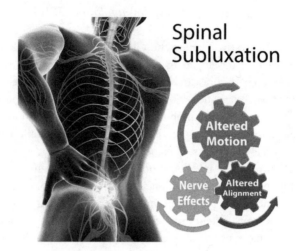

The DMR Method definition of Subluxation.

A subluxation is altered mobility or alignment of a joint that alters the normal mechanical function of a joint. It causes an imbalance in the nerves that control and coordinate local joint function and can cause imbalance in associated nerves that control and coordinated other areas of the body.

tissues improves. Phase two and three manipulations are often accompanied by an audible release of nitrogen gas that produces a "cracking" sound. Patients often experience some degree of relief immediately after a manipulation, but the real benefits are the long-term effects that Integrative Progressive Manipulations have on the reduction of subluxation and the restoration of mobility, alignment, and stability.

Chiropractors may use other therapies in conjunction with Integrated Progressive Manipulation such as electrical muscle stimulation, massage, traction, specific nutritional instruction, stretches, and exercises. These therapies enhance the effectiveness of IPM by treating the tissues surrounding the joints that are being manipulated.

Dynamic Muscle Technique (DMT)

Dynamic Muscle Technique is a three-phase system of hands-on soft-tissue mobilization and massage developed by the physical therapists involved in DMR Method development and research. DMT works in unison with other elements of DMR Method protocols to safely, comfortably, and efficiently

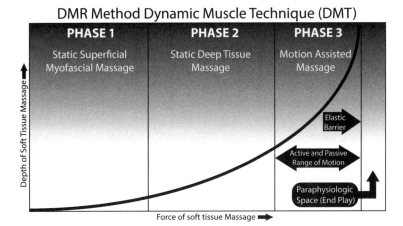

DMR Method Dynamic Muscle Technique (DMT)

decrease pain and spasm, and improve soft-tissue flexibility, healing, and reformation.

DMT is a progression that goes deeper into the supportive tissues with each phase. It is performed in synch with the three phases of Integrated Progressive Manipulation. The three phases of DMT include:

- *Phase One: Static Superficial Myofascial Mobilization*

  Static Superficial Myofascial Mobilization refers to the manual technique for stretching and mobilizing the fascia surrounding the muscles. Fascia is a seamless web of connective tissue that covers and connects the muscles, organs, and skeletal structures in the body. Injuries, stress, trauma, and poor posture can cause the fascia to become tight and inflamed. Because of the web-like structure of fascia, tightness in one part of the body can spread to other places in the body, much like pulling a thread in a piece of fabric can quickly destabilize other areas of the fabric. Fascia is the first layer of soft-tissue restriction and must be released before progressing deeper into the layers of supportive soft tissues. Static Superficial Myofascial Mobilization helps decrease pain, increase soft-tissue mobility, decrease muscle spasm, and improve lymphatic and blood circulation.

- *Phase Two: Static Deep-Tissue Massage*

  Static deep-tissue massage is generally more focused on specific muscles and muscle groups. In this phase of Dynamic Muscle Technique, your therapists access the deeper layers of soft tissue. Since each person experiences pressure differently, it's best to begin deep tissue massage by starting superficially and ease into the depth of the muscle slowly while carefully gauging sensitivity.. If the pressure is applied too deeply or too quickly, the muscle may tighten to protect that area, and unnecessary damage or inflammation can occur. Sometimes lubricant is used, depending on how far the pressure must travel over the skin. The benefits of Static Deep-Tissue Massage are similar to those of Static Superficial Myofascial Mobilization in phase one, but the effects are deeper and more localized.

- *Phase Three: Motion-Assisted Massage*

   Motion-assisted massage refers to the therapist using passive motion (the patient relaxes while the therapist moves a joint), or active motion (voluntary movement by the patient) during soft-tissue massage techniques. In many cases, this technique will help the mobility of the tissue being released, and will often help improve the patient's functional range of motion in the affected areas. When movement of the joints is performed during massage techniques, a reflexive relaxation occurs in the muscle group that opposes the motion being undertaken, which can also help to promote tissue release and improve subsequent flexibility efforts in that area.

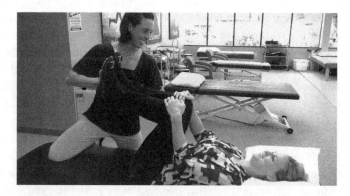

Spinal Traction

Spinal traction is not a new concept. Back in ancient times, people recognized the therapeutic value of "stretching the spine." Although the methods they employed back then are considered crude by today's standards, they often provided some benefit. Early traction methods ranged from hanging upside

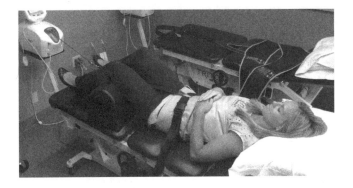

down from a tree to being strapped to a rack while ropes pulled the spine in opposite directions. Unfortunately, the idea of spinal traction remained on the fringe of healthcare until the National Aeronautic and Space Administration (NASA) began to do research on it.

More than a decade ago, astronauts began reporting that they experienced complete relief from back pain while in the zero-gravity environment of space. Researchers at NASA discovered why. When astronauts were in an anti-gravity state, the discs of their spine were not being compressed by gravity like they are on earth, allowing the discs to become fully hydrated and to reduce herniations (bulges) in the spinal discs. In fact, the fully hydrated discs resulted in many astronauts being two inches taller during their space flight. Because improved hydration of intervertebral discs can decrease severe back pain and improve the health of the spine, scientists were eager to reproduce the same effect here on earth.

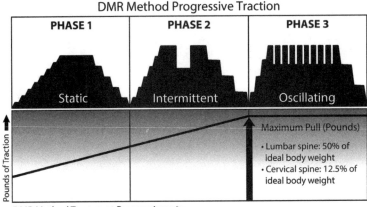

Spinal traction replicates an anti-gravity state and is used to mobilize discs and joints to encourage improved disc and joint hydration and mechanics. Essentially, spinal traction:

- helps restore motion to the affected joints;

- decreases pressure on the discs and stretches the supporting muscles and ligaments differently than other forms of mobilization and manipulation do;

- helps restore the hydrostatic pump mechanism which enhances joint and disc hydration;

- stimulates the nerve receptors (proprioceptors) in the joints and surrounding muscles and ligaments responsible for enhancing posture, alignment, and coordination.

Standard medically excepted traction procedures are used in a specific progression. Because the effects of traction are beneficial throughout treatment it's typically used in all three phases of the DMR Method.

Cold Laser Therapy

Cold laser therapy is an effective treatment option for a wide range of acute and chronic conditions. Cold laser therapy has three primary advantages. First, it is extremely safe. Because no heat is generated by the laser, there is virtually no risk of damaging the tissues you are trying to heal. This is especially important in acute injuries where the tissues are inflamed and swollen, because applying heat (as ultrasound and other methods do) could make the inflammation worse.

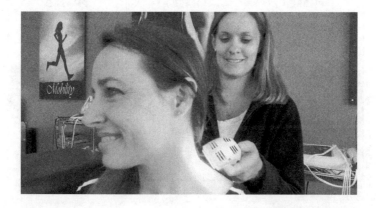

Second, unlike medications that travel throughout the body and frequently lead to side effects, cold laser therapy is applied directly to the affected area. This not only focuses and concentrates all the therapeutic power specifically to the affected area, it also eliminates the risk of side effects.

Third, cold laser light actually stimulates tissue regeneration at the cellular level. Where other forms of therapy simply decrease pain or inflammation, cold laser therapy works at the cellular level to stimulate the mitochondria within the cells to produce ATP, the fuel for the cell. Increased levels of ATP allow the cells to work more quickly to repair damaged tissues, resulting in quicker healing times.

A Note About Medications and Injections

Sometimes medications and/or injections may be necessary to aid in recovery by helping control symptoms and inflammation. At the same time, many prescription drugs, particularly pain medication, may help you feel better by masking the symptoms of a problem area in your body while not doing anything to fix the problem itself. DMR Method providers work alongside medical pain specialists, orthopedists, neurologists, neurosurgeons, and general practitioners to help make each patient's recovery as efficient as possible. A medical consultation may be included in your program to determine if any additions or changes should be made to any medications you may be taking in order to aid in your recovery. Sometimes, persistent symptoms or inflammation can prevent a normal DMR Method progression; in such cases, a diagnostic or therapeutic injection consultation may be recommended.

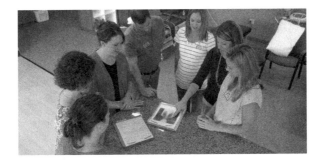

Coordinating Care

As you can see, the DMR Method includes many different components, all of which work together synergistically to relieve symptoms and correct the cause of those symptoms by restoring mobility, alignment, and stability.

It's crucial that the right components are synchronized with each other at the right time, in the right order, with the right intensity, for the right duration. This truly is the "secret sauce" of the DMR Method and the reason why it's proven so successful for so many people.

In the next chapter, we'll take a closer look at the DMR Method treatment program and help you get started on your road to recovery.

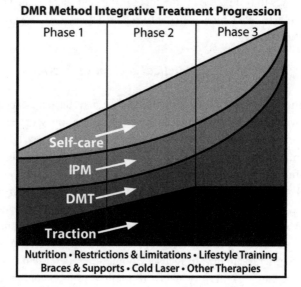

DMR Method Integrative Treatment Progression

Combining the right components of treatment at the right time, in the right order, with the right intensity, for the right duration is hallmark of the DMR Method

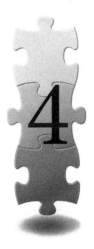

Your DMR Program

So far we've described the anatomy of the spine, what can go wrong, the three keys to treating spinal conditions, the three phases of the recovery process, and the elements that comprise the DMR Method treatment protocol. Now it's time to pull all that information together to present the DMR Method treatment program. The program is organized in both a descriptive and a practical way so patients can refer back to this chapter to understand, organize, and track their own personal DMR Method treatment program.

Before Your Initial Consultation

Before you come in for an initial DMR Method consultation, here are five things you can do to make the process go more smoothly:

- First, gather any previous medical records together—especially X-rays, MRI scans, and any other diagnostic test results. Lists of medications and supplements are also helpful.

- Second, review the history of your condition and make note of any treatments, flare-ups, setbacks, injuries, or other occurrences that may have impacted your recovery in some way. No item is too small to mention.

- Third, Go to DMRmethod.com and click on "Patient Resources," then "Patient Forms" and fill out the Patient Intake form. If you have a neck condition, fill out the Neck Disability Index form. If you have a lower back condition, fill out the Oswestry Disability Index form.

- Fourth, familiarize yourself with the DMR Method. Reading this book is the best way to do that, but visiting DMRmethod.com and watching the educational and testimonial videos is also helpful. While many patients have already experienced one or more components (chiropractic, physical therapy, traction, etc.) of the DMR Method with other healthcare providers, remember that the DMR Method is a structured process of evaluation and treatment. The order of each component and the manner in which they're combined are critical to a successful outcome. The more that patients know, the more they will understand the importance of each step and the more they will be able to constructively participate in their care. In addition, taking a video tour of the DMR Method treatment facility will help you become familiar with the clinical setting.

- Fifth, attitude is everything. Many patients have become frustrated after trying so many approaches that have proved ineffective. Examinations, diagnostic testing, medications, injections, therapy, chiropractic, more testing—the list goes on and on. In fact, many patients who come to our clinic are suffering from depression due to their ongoing pain and disability. So before you come in for your initial consultation, it can be helpful to tell yourself that you are starting anew with a protocol that is more innovative and organized than anything you've done before. The right attitude can help you become a more active and engaged participant in your recovery process.

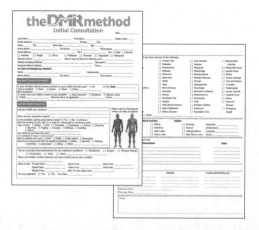

The Initial Consultation form can be found on our website:
www.DMRmethod.com/Patient-Resources/Patient-Forms/

The Keys to Success!

1. Be informed- Understand everything about your condition and the recommended treatment.

2. Follow your DMR treatment protocol- including restrictions, nutrition, stretching, exercises, clinical care and appropriate maintenance care. Do it all, and in the right order.

3. Let you DMR providers guide you- They've treated thousands of patients like you and will keep you on track and make the right modifications to your treatment when necessary.

4. Be involved- You are the most important participant in your recovery. Do everything you're supposed to and be consistent.

5. Follow through- Even when you feel and function better, keep following your treatment protocol to assure your body has enough time to heal completely. Treat the condition, not the symptoms.

The Initial Consultation: Forming the Team

We begin the DMR Method initial consultation by discussing your condition with you (and, if you'd like, your spouse or other loved one). This is an important step because it not only helps us understand the physical issues you're dealing with, it gives us insight into your state of mind and attitude. Remember, the DMR Method treatment process requires commitment from a team of healthcare providers and the patient, so the patient needs to be a willing and active member of the team right from the start. Amazingly, many patients who initially feel hopeless, unwilling, or even skeptical end up being some of the best team players and attain incredible life-changing results.

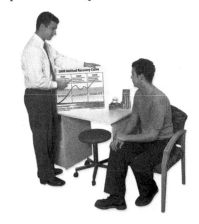

The DMR Method Initial Consultation form, which is filled out prior to or at the time of the first appointment, is used as a guide for the evaluating clinician to conduct a focused and constructive consultation. The consultation form is also designed to help you begin thinking broadly about your condition so that the evaluating clinician gains as much information as possible about how it's impacting your life.

The objectives of the DMR Method initial consultation are to:

- gain in-depth knowledge about you and your condition;
- identify the onset of your condition;
- determine the quality and grade of your symptoms;
- determine the timing and pattern of symptoms (local or radiating?);
- identify what makes your symptoms worse or better;
- gather information about your treatment history;
- learn about your lifestyle habits;
- identify what supplements and medications you're taking;
- gather information about your medical and family history;
- review your pain and disability indexes, which evaluate how your current condition is affecting your life.

We also review your previous medical records during the initial consultation. This review may include previous evaluation and treatment records and previous diagnostic imaging, including X-rays, CT/MRI scans, or other special imaging. The more medical records you can provide the better; they deepen our understanding of your condition and guide us toward any additional testing that may need to be done.

The Examination: Finding the True Cause of Your Condition

The initial consultation enables us to identify a focus for the DMR Method examination, which is a structured and standardized process. The examination is designed to help us determine if you are a candidate for the DMR Method. Remember, it's just as important to identify those we can't help as those we can so that we can make appropriate recommendations and referrals if necessary. Once the examination is complete, we will be equipped to accurately diagnosis your condition and prescribe which specific DMR Method protocol to follow for optimal results.

Your Initial Visit Checklist

Your checklist of things to do:

☐ *Gather your previous records, including diagnostic imaging and other test results.*

☐ *Review the history of your condition.*

☐ *Fill out the Patient Intake form and the appropriate Disability Index forms at DMRMethod.com/Patient-Resources/Patient-Forms*

☐ *Learn about the DMR Method by reading this book and exploring the DMRMethod.com website.*

☐ *Cultivate a positive, hopeful attitude that your condition can be resolved and you will be able to resume all of your normal activities.*

Notes:

_____

_____

_____

Questions You Would Like to Ask:

_____

_____

_____

_____

Forms may be downloaded at our website at:
www.DMRMethod.com/Patient-Resources/Patient-Forms

A typical DMR Method examination looks at several key areas:

- Vital Signs

- Posture Analysis

- Neurological Testing

- Range of Motion Testing

- Orthopedic Testing

- Palpation (feeling with hands)

- Muscle tonicity/spasm/tenderness

- Joint position/symmetry

- Joint motion

- Diagnostic Testing

- X-rays

- MRI Referral

- Other Diagnostic Testing (Lab work/neurological/nutritional)

Tips for Your Initial Examination

☐ *Wear comfortable clothes; avoid wearing items that are difficult to remove (panty hose, zip-up dress, multiple layers of clothing, pants with suspenders).*

☐ *Avoid wearing jewelry.*

☐ *If you have long hair, bring clips or binders to put your hair up.*

☐ *Make sure you're as comfortable as possible. Your symptoms may not be changeable, but make sure to eliminate any uncomfortable factors that you can control. If you have to go to the restroom, if you're too hot or too cold, or if you need some water, let your DMR Method practitioner or one of the assistants know and they'll do everything they can to make you comfortable.*

☐ *Relax. The examination is nothing to be nervous about. In fact, for many it marks the beginning of the end of a painful, stressful condition.*

☐ *Ask questions. You should understand every step in the DMR Method Evaluation and Treatment process.*

Your Diagnosis

Following the consultation and examination, your practitioner will review the findings and present a diagnosis. Even if you've seen many different healthcare providers for your condition, this diagnosis may be different than anything you've previously been told. Certainly, if you have a condition like a disc herniation, stenosis, or degenerative disc disease, that element would be consistent among providers. But it's important to differentiate the symptoms of your condition from the cause of your condition. Your treatment program focuses on treating the cause of your condition, which almost always can be traced to deficiencies in mobility, alignment, and stability.

Your DMR Method Program: DMR Diagnosis

Conditions:

_____

_____

Causes:

_____

_____

_____

Knowledge is power! Make sure you thoroughly understand your condition and the causes of your condition. Your practitioner has numerous resources to help answer any questions you may have.

The Treatment Plan: Creating Your Game Plan

Your treatment plan will be formulated in a way that is most appropriate for your particular condition based on the results of your initial consultation, examination, and diagnosis. As we discuss in the case studies throughout this book, each patient follows a specific protocol of care based on the unique circumstances of their condition. So don't be surprised if your treatment plan differs somewhat from the plans of other people with similar conditions.

The DMR Method Patient Guidebook is typically used as a template to design your treatment program. You may also use this guidebook as a quick reference to your treatment plan and schedule of care. It will also give you step-by-step instructions for what you need to do on your own to optimize your recovery.

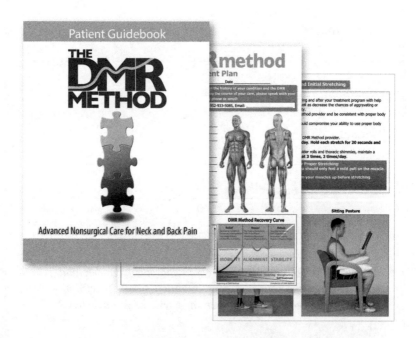

The DMR Method Patient Guidebook is a resource to help you organize all the components of you DMR Method program. It includes key symptoms, exam findings, your diagnosis, treatment recommendations, nutritional, self-care, exercise and stretching guidelines as well as recovery goals.

The DMR Method Treatment Progression:
It's All About Teamwork

Starting from day one, specific elements of care, goals, and education will be addressed every visit. The collaborative process between the patient, physical therapist, chiropractor and allied medical providers, and the synergistic role each plays in the progression of care, is essential to achieve favorable outcomes.

Amy's Story

I am an avid runner and speed walker. After having finished my ninth week of physical therapy at another clinic and not seeing ANY improvement, I was told I should see a spine surgeon to discuss medication and possible surgery. My husband and I decided that we would keep trying natural ways of treating my herniated disc until there were no options left but surgery.

My father-in-law mentioned an advertisement he saw for a special treatment for herniated discs called the DMR Method. I was extremely skeptical that the ten-week DMR Method treatment would be able to relieve my sciatic nerve pain from a herniated disc. However, we decided to give it a shot.

It was about three weeks into my treatment when my husband told me my leg must be feeling better because he hadn't heard me complain about pain for a while. My physical therapist asked me each morning how I was feeling and each time I'd tell her that everything felt great, but I still didn't know how speed walking or running would affect me.

Towards the end of the ten weeks, my physical therapist said that the only way we'd know if I was healed was to try walking and then running. I went to the gym that night and started with five minutes of speed walking on the treadmill and felt no pain whatsoever! From there we increased the time and speed until I was running for thirty minutes without pain.

I am extremely impressed with the attention and care I was given and would recommend to anyone suffering from back pain to give the DMR Method a chance. Now I laugh when I think that I even considered surgery because this treatment got rid of my pain in less than ten weeks without surgery or scars.

-Amy F.

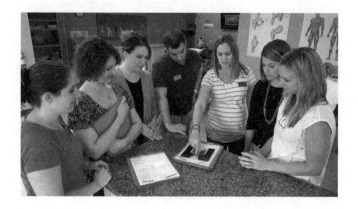

To illustrate this idea, let's say you want to cook a chicken breast. You light a match and wave it under the meat until it burns out. The chicken may have gotten a little warm but the match was largely ineffective. Even if you light match after match under the chicken until it's thoroughly cooked or you run out of matches, you've spent a lot of time on something that may or may not be successful. Now, let's say you have that same book of matches but you also have some charcoal and lighter fluid. If you pile up the charcoal just right, add some lighter fluid, then light it with a match, you can cook the chicken breast and enjoy the benefits of your barbecue in just a few minutes. The right components in the right order produce superior—and delicious—results!

Implementing the right components in the right order is what makes the DMR Method treatment progression so unique and successful. Its development required years of research and countless hours of work "in the trenches" by a dedicated team of physical therapists, chiropractors, and medical doctors. As mentioned in chapter 3, this effort produced a graduated system of spinal manipulation called Integrated Progressive Manipulation, a specific progression of soft-tissue therapy called Dynamic Muscle Technique and a unique sequence of spinal traction called DMR Method Progressive Traction. Individually, each technique is effective. What makes these three modalities groundbreaking is how they reinforce each other through a progression of care to maximize safety, improve effectiveness, and accelerate the speed of recovery.

This unique synergistic method of treatment is evident from the very beginning of treatment when your treatment team starts the process of restoring motion to the affected joints. To do this, they will begin the first phase of Dynamic Muscle Technique, Integrated Progressive Manipulation and Progressive traction simultaneously. As mobility begins to improve, they progress to phase two of each modality. This cooperative procedure progresses through a third and final phase at which time joint motion is restored to maximum potential.

However, IPM, DMT, and Progressive Traction are only three components of the DMR Method treatment progression. Other components are simultaneously taking place that are also essential to a full recovery.

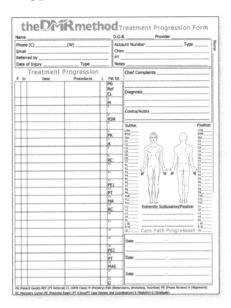

The physical therapists and chiropractors use the Treatment Progression Form as an outline to follow and as a tool to track progress. They will provide you with all the resources you need to participate in your recovery.

The DMR Method Treatment Protocols

Given that the circumstances of each patient's condition are unique, treatment protocols are customized based upon the diagnosis, how long a patient has had the condition, how old the patient is, whether the patient has had surgery, and other factors.

We start by identifying a general protocol of care and then adapting that protocol to each individual's needs. During the course of care, the protocol may need to be adjusted depending on the patient's response to treatment. The goal of your DMR Method practitioner is to progress you through the relief, repair, and rehab phases of the DMR Method as efficiently as possible and attain the goals of symptom relief, functional improvement, and restored mobility, alignment, and stability.

There are three main DMR Method treatment protocols: the Limited Protocol, the Progressed Protocol, and the Advanced Protocol. While there are many factors that determine which protocol is best for a particular patient, the two main determining factors are the severity of the patient's condition and the amount of time the patient has had the condition. Let's take a look at each of these protocols and how each one is used.

Clinical Care Protocol Algorithm

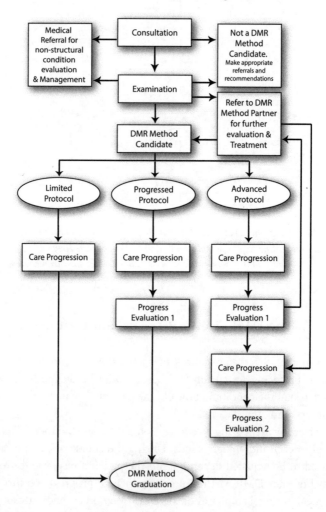

Limited Protocol

The DMR Method Limited Protocol is for recent, less severe conditions. Examples include minor strain/sprain injuries, most sports injuries, back and neck stiffness, tension headaches, and acute facet joint syndrome. Only a limited number of the DMR Method treatment elements are necessary and patients progress rapidly through the three phases of recovery (relief, repair, rehab). Patients are then transitioned to self-care. Treatment is typically completed in four to six weeks over four to twelve visits.

Progressed Protocol

The DMR Method Progressed Protocol (commonly referred to as the "normal" protocol) is appropriate for moderate conditions of longer duration. Examples include moderate strain/sprain and sports injuries and non-radiating persistent back and neck pain. Not all of the DMR Method treatment elements are necessary, and there is typically a focus on Integrated Progressive Manipulation (IPM), Dynamic Muscle Technique (DMT), and a targeted stretching and exercise program. Patients typically progress through the three phases of recovery (relief, repair, rehab) in four to eight weeks over twelve to twenty visits.

Advanced Protocol

The DMR Method Advanced Protocol was developed for severe conditions of both short-term and long-term duration. Examples include severe strain/sprain injures with ligamentous instability, disc herniations, sciatica, stenosis, degenerative disc disease, slippage conditions in the spine (spondylolisthesis), and failed back surgery syndrome. Most, if not all, of the DMR Method treatment elements are necessary, and close clinical monitoring and case management is necessary in the first phase of recovery. Patients typically progress though the three phases of recovery (relief, repair, rehab) in ten to twelve weeks over twenty to twenty-four visits and may require some periodic follow-up care.

Note: All of the patients who had pre- and post-MRI scans done in the DMR Method case studies were treated with the DMR Method Advanced Protocol because they all had conditions that were identifiable and measurable on MRI scans.

Which DMR Method Protocol is Right for You?

DMR Method practitioners carefully review all the information gathered during the consultation and examination to determine which DMR Method protocol is appropriate for each patient. They then decide which elements of the protocol are necessary and where to place the most focus in order to move patients through the three phases of recovery as efficiently as possible.

Your Treatment Protocol

A great deal of effort goes into the process of evaluating your condition and identifying the right course of care to follow. Your DMR Method practitioner will sit down with you and explain which protocol of treatment is recommended or, if you are not a candidate for the DMR Method, what course of care would be more appropriate. Be sure to ask your practitioner questions until you thoroughly understand all the elements of your treatment plan.

Your Treatment Progression

The right clinical care protocol for your diagnosis is established by your consultation and evaluation. Although every case is unique, there are certain aspects, landmarks, and goals that are common throughout the progression of care. Once the your treatment progression begins, your providers follow the DMR Method Treatment Algorithm and use the DMR Method Recovery Curve to assure that you stay on course.

Review of the DMR Recovery Curve

Another important treatment tool is the recovery curve, which has three specific phases. Understanding these phases will help you and your providers track your progress and make any changes necessary to keep your recovery on course.

The DMR Method recovery curve shows how your symptoms and functional abilities should improve during the course of treatment. The curve was created by tracking thousands of DMR Method cases. Most patients follow a symptomatic and functional recovery close to the one illustrated in the graphic below. Let's take a moment to review the highlights of these three recovery phases:

DMR Method Treatment Algorithm

The Relief Phase

During the relief phase, you should feel symptoms improve rapidly. More challenging cases may require six to nine treatments before symptoms begin to resolve. Symptom relief is due to decreased inflammation and improved mobility. As your symptoms dramatically decrease, you may feel the urge to resume normal physical activity; however, it's important to follow the restrictions given to you by your DMR Method practitioner.

Your DMR Method Program: Treatment Plan

Recommended DMR Method Protocol:

_____

Special Instructions:

_____

_____

_____

Keys to Recovery:

_____

_____

_____

Questions / Notes:

_____

_____

_____

_____

_____

Remember: Use your DMR Method Patient Guidebook from the very beginning of your treatment program. It summarizes your case and gives you everything you need to understand the clinical and self-care components of your treatment.

The Repair Phase

During the repair phase, your symptoms will continue to improve although they may fluctuate slightly, and you will begin to experience improvements in your physical abilities. Your body has begun the process of repairing and reforming the supportive soft tissues surrounding the affected area. This is the phase in which actual healing of the condition begins. Even so, your symptoms may fluctuate for two reasons.

First, when you feel better—especially when you haven't known what it feels like to be free of pain in a long time—you may stop performing the self-care procedures necessary for recovery. You may also start doing physical activities that are too aggressive or outside your restrictions. The joints and supportive soft tissues that were immobile are often weak, deconditioned, and not ready for increased physical activity.

Second, sensory nerves in joints (called proprioceptors) that have been "turned off" due to lack of motion are suddenly "turned on" again (which is a good thing because you need those nerves to help direct coordination and alignment of the joints). Although this is essential for correction, it temporally creates instability because the sensory nerves in the joints have to essentially relearn how to control and coordinate joint function and balance.

In the repair phase, the joints, supportive soft tissue, and sensory nerves are in a state of transition. They're no longer in the condition they used to be, but they're not yet in the condition they're supposed to be. It's crucial to stay consistent with all elements of the repair phase of treatment. The more you do, the fewer bumps in the road you'll have to contend with.

The Rehab Phase

The rehab phase is the most important phase of the DMR Method. You've put a lot of effort into restoring mobility and alignment and getting the healing process started. You will now begin the process of stabilizing your condition, the key to long-term management and lasting results. In the rehab phase, your symptoms will be resolved to their maximum potential and no longer fluctuate, your physical abilities will be restored, and your treatment will shift from clinical care to self-care. You'll learn advanced stretching and strengthening techniques, and how to maintain your recovery with proper body mechanics and appropriate restrictions. At the end of the rehab phase, you'll graduate from the clinical treatment portion of the DMR Method and have a clear understanding of what you need to do on your own to ensure excellent health and well-being going forward.

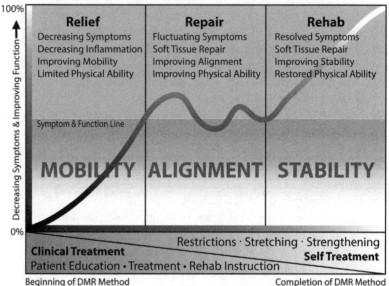

The DMR Method Recovery Curve

100%

↑ Decreasing Symptoms & Improving Function

Relief
Decreasing Symptoms
Decreasing Inflammation
Improving Mobility
Limited Physical Ability

Repair
Fluctuating Symptoms
Soft Tissue Repair
Improving Alignment
Improving Physical Ability

Rehab
Resolved Symptoms
Soft Tissue Repair
Improving Stability
Restored Physical Ability

Symptom & Function Line

MOBILITY   ALIGNMENT   STABILITY

0%

Restrictions · Stretching · Strengthening
Clinical Treatment   **Self Treatment**
Patient Education • Treatment • Rehab Instruction

Beginning of DMR Method   Completion of DMR Method

Tracking Your Progress

Throughout your DMR Method treatment progression, it's important that you and your practitioner track your progress. Knowing what to expect at each stage of your recovery will help you monitor your progress more confidently and understand the importance of the self-care elements that will be introduced during the various stages of recovery. Your DMR Method provider team treats thousands of cases per year; that experience helps them quickly identify when a course correction needs to be made to keep your recovery on track.

The DMR Method treatment progression chart on page 76 displays all the different elements of clinical treatment and self-care and when they are typically introduced. It also shows the frequency of clinical treatment, the phases of care, and the goal of each phase. Remember, every DMR Method treatment plan is individualized, so the components and timing may vary in order to maximize the benefits and speed of recovery.

You can track your recovery on the personal recovery curve on the following page. Mark on the scale that reflects your symptoms and functionality after each visit. Check each self-care component when it has been implemented. If you have unusual symptoms or disability, make note of it and speak to your provider about it as soon as possible.

Your DMR Method Program: Track Your Recovery

Track your recovery on your personal recovery curve below. Mark on the scale where you're at symptomatically and functionally after each visit. Check off each self-care component when it has been implemented. If you have fluctuating symptoms or disability, write what you did or didn't do that may have been a contributing factor in the space below the scale. Note: If you don't feel like your following a typical recovery curve, make sure to speak to your provider immediately.

Relief
O Strict Restrictions
O Basic Body Mechanics
O Supportive Nutrition
O Braces/Supports
O Light Stretching
Other: _____
_____

Repair
O Moderate Restrictions
O Progressed Body Mechanics
O Advanced Stretching
O Static Exercises
Other: _____
_____

Rehab
O Light Restrictions
O Dynamic Exercises
O Personalized Self-Care Program
Other: _____

Symptom & Function Line

MOBILITY ALIGNMENT STABILITY

Day: 1 2 3 4 5 6 7 8 9 10 11 12 13 14 15 16 17 18 19 20 21 22 23 24

Notes:

_____
_____
_____
_____
_____
_____

DMR Method Graduation

Congratulations, you have just completed a groundbreaking and systematic process of evaluation and treatment. Both you and your DMR Method practitioner have worked hard. Now it's time for you to take the reins and continue the process of getting your body stronger and more stable. You may have made incredible progress in a short period of time and feel like you have finally gotten ahead of your condition, but it's important at this point to differentiate between short-term symptom relief and long-term healing. The eleven-to-eighteen-month rule can help you make that distinction.

The Eleven-to-Eighteen-Month Rule

Depending upon which DMR Method treatment protocol you followed, your course of care lasted between four and twelve weeks, and at the end of your treatment your DMR Method practitioner gave you instructions on what to do on your own and, if necessary, when to come back in for a check-up. Your practitioner also explained that even though you're feeling much better, you need to continue with consistent self-care and follow any restrictions you may have been given for eleven to eighteen months. This time frame is based on the knowledge that the ligaments that provide structural support and stability to your joints take many months, or even years, to heal completely. Inside that time, they are vulnerable to re-injury. This particular range of time was arrived at for a number of reasons; age, activity level, nutrition, genetics, and other factors all play a role in how fast your ligaments will heal.

From a structural, functional, and neurological basis, the ligaments that support your joints need to be as healthy and strong as possible. Therefore, we strongly recommend that you stay consistent with all your self-care

Damaged Ligament   *Normal Ligament*

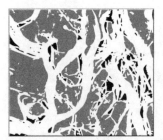 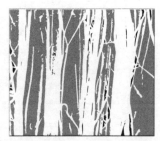

Repair of damages ligaments takes 11-18 months to heal if managed correctly.

procedures and restrictions for at least eleven to eighteen months following your graduation from the clinical treatment portion of your DMR Method Program.

DMR Method Maintenance Care

Maintenance care includes everything you do to ensure and enhance your recovery. By far, the most important maintenance care involves the activities you do on your own. These self-care procedures include proper body mechanics, pacing your physical activity, stretching, exercise, healthy nutrition, and managing any physical restrictions. Your DMR Method practitioner has provided you with all the instruction and resources you need; if you need further guidance, feel free to contact your practitioner at any time.

Remember, it's essential that you stay consistent with all your maintenance care procedures, especially in the first eleven to eighteen months. That may sound like a long time, but when you consider the effort you've already put into your recovery, how much better you feel, and your improved ability to be physically active, you'll appreciate the value of sticking with your maintenance care. Your personal program was designed specifically for your unique circumstances, will take minimal time each day, and will make you feel great!

Maintenance care may also include some forms of treatment that you can't do on your own but are still essential after you've completed your treatment program. These may include periodic Integrated Progressive Manipulation, Dynamic Muscle Technique, Oscillating Decompression Traction (ODT), or other skilled treatment that will help maintain your recovery. Your DMR Method practitioner's goal is to help you do everything that you can on your own; but when clinical maintenance care is necessary, your practitioner will tell you what you need to do and how often you need to do it. Some cases progress to a point where the patient's symptoms have resolved and their physical abilities are improved, but due to the nature of their condition a core structural problem persists. In these cases, patients may benefit from proactively receiving specific forms of skilled maintenance treatment on a regular basis. For example, a patient with severe degenerative disc disease may benefit from a short series of traction treatments once a year to help maintain core joint and disc mobility.

Your DMR Method Program:
Maintenance Care Quick Reference

In chapter five, Self-Care & Exercise Guide, there's a complete instruction guide for all the self-care procedures that will help you maintain your recovery. It's organized in different categories of self-care. You can use this book as your one stop resource for all self-care procedures. All you have to do is take the self-care reference sheets given to you by your provider and write the number of each treatment procedure in the appropriate category below. Just go to the procedure number on the top of the page in chapter five and you'll have all the instruction you need to stay consistent. If you need help organizing this, make sure to ask your DMR Method provider and they'll be happy to assist you.

Lifestyle Training:

B: _____

Stretching:

S: _____

Stabilizing Exercises:

E: _____

Proprioceptive Training Exercises:

P: _____

Super Sets:

SS: _____

Questions / Notes:

_____

DMR Method™ Case Study

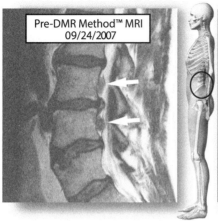
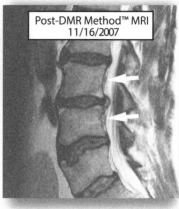

Pre-DMR Method™ MRI
09/24/2007

Post-DMR Method™ MRI
11/16/2007

Multiple Disc Herniations Lumbar Spine

John developed severe debilitating lower back pain after lifting improperly. His pain continued for weeks and worsened after doing housework, radiating down his left leg. He couldn't stand without leaning forward and his leg felt weak and unstable.

DIAGNOSIS

An MRI scan revealed two large herniations between L4-5 and L3-4 in the lumbar spine causing left-sided nerve root impingement. DMR Method Evaluation revealed severe spinal immobility in the lumbar spine and pelvis, muscle and ligament remodeling and lower back and pelvic misalignment, causing excessive pressure on the lower lumbar discs.

TREATMENT

Acute Lumbar DMR Protocol for multiple herninations that included a lumbar support belt and strict limitations on physical activities to prevent aggravation or re-injury.

OUTCOME

Complete resolution of back and leg symptoms and a return to normal physical activity. A follow-up MRI eight weeks after the initial MRI revealed reabsorption of L4-5 and L3-4 disc herniations. His seven-year follow-up confirmed continued symptom resolution and normal to enhanced physical abilities.

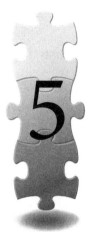

Self-Care and
Exercise Guide

A common misconception among patients is that their body will be able to heal itself as long as they keep all their appointments. Of course, that implies that all the therapy their body needs can be condensed into a couple of short visits per week.

The therapy provided during your clinic visits is indeed vital to your recovery, but what you do between visits is equally as important. Hours upon hours of poor posture, lifting incorrectly, poor diet, and stress can neutralize the cumulative effect of all the various therapies performed during clinic visits. A full recovery from an injury requires a long-term lifestyle change.

Think about someone who goes to a gym to improve their health and lose weight. If they followed up each workout with a trip to a fast-food restaurant to eat a super-sized meal full of fat and sugar, they'd be sabotaging their weight-loss goals. The same principle holds true for someone recovering from an injury.

The following pages include a guide for how to perform everyday activities in a way that minimizes the stress on your body. You'll also find a series of therapeutic exercises and stretches that your physical therapist or doctor will instruct you to do. Don't worry, you won't have to do all of them. Depending on your particular situation, you may be given anywhere from one to several exercises and stretches to do at home between clinic visits to help facilitate the quickest recovery possible.

How to Use this Guide

Everything you need to do to assist in your recovery is contained in this chapter. Each group of activities is important. Your DMR Method provider will design your personal self-care program by selecting the right procedures for you to follow in each of the categories below. The tabs at the top of each page will help make your self-care program as user-friendly as possible. The procedures are organized into six basic groups:

- **Restrictions and Physical Limitations**

  These essential restrictions and limitations will help prevent aggravation and re-injury

- **Lifestyle Training**

  Learning proper techniques will minimize the impact that normal daily activities will have on your condition

- **Stretching**

  These specific stretching techniques are designed to improve the mobility of the affected joints, muscles, and ligaments

- **Exercises**

  This progression of exercises will improve strength, stability, and coordination

- **Balance Exercises**

  These advanced exercises will enhance stability, coordination, and proprioception

- **Super Sets**

  These quick five-minute workouts include stretching, strengthening, and balancing elements to help you stay consistent with your self-care program no matter where you are

Note: Do not begin any of the following procedures without the guidance and instruction of your DMR Method provider.

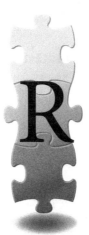

Restrictions and Physical Limitations

When you begin your treatment program, one of the first things your provider will do is define appropriate restrictions and physical limitations. These instructions for work or at home will help prevent aggravation or re-injury and help you progress as rapidly as possible. Your provider may also recommend that you use a specific brace, support, or other tool. It's important that you follow these recommendations throughout your recovery, and that you adhere to any restrictions and limitations as your symptoms begin to resolve. Remember, even though you may feel remarkably better, your body has a lot of healing to do and it's essential that you give your body the time it needs to heal. Honoring your restrictions and limitations will maximize the speed and extent of your recovery.

Physical Restrictions

☐   *Sedentary. Lifting ten pounds maximum and occasionally lifting and/or carrying such articles as dockets, ledgers, small tools, and household items. Although sedentary physical activity is defined as primarily sitting, occasional walking and standing is often necessary to carry out daily activities.*

☐   *Light Physical Activity. Lifting twenty pounds maximum with frequent lifting and/or carrying of objects weighing up to ten pounds. Even though the weight lifted may be a negligible amount, physical activity can include a significant degree of walking or standing. Light physical activity can also include sitting most of the time while pushing and pulling with your arms and/or leg controls.*

☐   *Medium Physical Activity. Lifting fifty pounds maximum with frequent lifting and/or carrying of objects weighing up to twenty-five pounds.*

☐   *Heavy Physical Activity. Lifting seventy-five pounds maximum with frequent lifting and/or carrying of object weighing up to forty pounds.*

☐   *Very Heavy Physical Activity. Lifting one hundred pounds maximum with frequent lifting and/or carrying of objects weighing fifty pounds.*

Notes: _____

_____

_____

_____

_____

_____

_____

_____

Physical Limitations

1. **In a day, patient may:**

   A. Stand/Walk
   - ☐ None   ☐ 4-6 Hours   ☐ 1-4 Hours
   - ☐ 6-8 Hours
   - ☐ Other: _____

   B. Sit
   - ☐ 1-3 Hours   ☐ 3-5 Hours   ☐ 5-8 Hours
   - ☐ Other: _____

   C. Drive
   - ☐ 1-3 Hours   ☐ 3-5 Hours   ☐ 5-8 Hours
   - ☐ Other: _____

2. Patient may use hands for repetitive:
   - ☐ Single Grasping   ☐ Pushing & Pulling
   - ☐ Fine Manipulation

3. Patient may use feet for repetitive movement, as in operating foot controls:
   - ☐ Yes   ☐ No

4. Patient is able to:

	Frequently	Occasionally	Not at all
a. Bend	☐	☐	☐
b. Bend & Twist	☐	☐	☐
c. Climb	☐	☐	☐
d. Kneel	☐	☐	☐
e. Reaching Overhead	☐	☐	☐

Other: _____

_____

_____

_____

_____

Braces, Supports and Other Tools

Your DMR Method provider may recommend that you use a specific brace, support, or other adaptive tool to assist in your recovery. These recommendations are designed to protect, support, and decrease undue stress on your body. Examples of these tools include:

- Lumbar support belts
- Cervical collars
- Heel lifts
- Kinesiotaping
- Orthopedic pillows
- Lumbar-support chair cushion
- Book stands or other ergonomic tools
- Sacroiliac stability belt

Your provider will make appropriate recommendations and give you detailed instructions on how to implement these tools as needed into your treatment program.

How to Put on a Lumbar Brace

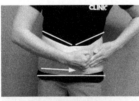
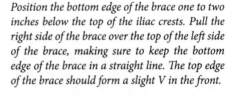

Position the bottom edge of the brace one to two inches below the top of the iliac crests. Pull the right side of the brace over the top of the left side of the brace, making sure to keep the bottom edge of the brace in a straight line. The top edge of the brace should form a slight V in the front.

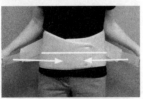

Simultaneously pull both secondary elastic straps around to the front and attach the velcro tabs below the midline on the brace.

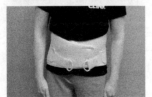

This is the way the lumbosacral corset brace should look when it's put on properly.

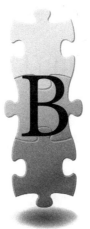

Lifestyle Training

When performing daily physical activities, using proper body mechanics is another way to decrease stress on the area being treated. Just like your restrictions and physical limitations, proper body mechanics will help expedite your recovery and prevent the chances of aggravating or re-injuring your condition. Because it takes eleven to eighteen months for the supportive soft tissues in your body to reach full strength, it's essential that you continue to use proper body mechanics on an ongoing basis.

B1

Standing Posture

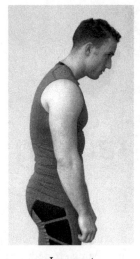 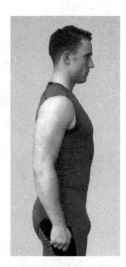

Incorrect   *Correct*

- Stand with weight equally borne on feet (avoid leaning too heavily on one side)
- Have feet positioned so they face forward
- Draw your head back so that it is centered as closely as possible over your shoulders
- Relax your scapulae and bring them downward and toward each other to support your upper back
- Slightly tighten your abdominal muscles by bringing your belly button closer to your spine
- Keep knees relaxed—not locked into hyperextension—while standing

Quick Tip: Push the top of your head straight up as though you are trying to elongate your body, then relax slightly.

Sitting Posture

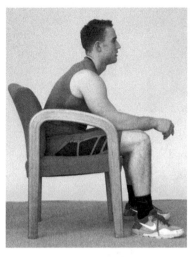 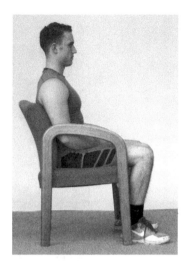

Incorrect   *Correct*

- Make sure both feet are flat on the floor, with ankles uncrossed

- Your hips and knees should be at 90-degree angles

- Your head should be over your hips (not forward of your shoulders)

- Use a pillow or towel in the small of your lumbar spine to support that area

- Keep your abdominal muscles engaged to support lumbar curvature

Quick Tip: From a seated position with your feet flat on the floor, push the top of your head straight up as though you are trying to elongate your body, then relax slightly.

Getting Into Bed

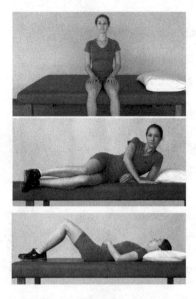

- Position yourself so your back faces the middle of the bed

- Slowly bend at the knees and hips, keeping your spine straight

- Use your hands to feel the surface of the bed and to help lower yourself into a seated position

- Using your arm closest to the head of the bed, lower your upper trunk toward the pillow, keeping your head and spine in line; as you begin to lean, swing your legs up onto the bed, taking care not to twist your trunk as you do so

- Once your legs are supported by the bed, lower your upper trunk toward the pillow, and lay your head on the pillow without turning your head; your spine should be in a straight line while lying on your side

- From this position, you can slowly adjust yourself to allow for greater comfort

Getting Out of Bed

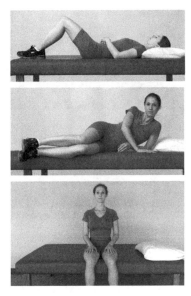

- Bend your knees so your feet are together
- Perform a pelvic tilt by pulling your belly button toward your spine to engage your abdominal muscles
- Push downward with your feet to lift your buttocks off the bed slightly, allowing you to shift your body closer to the edge of the bed
- Keeping your knees bent and your spine in line, roll as a unit until you are lying on your side
- Bend your bottom arm to allow your elbow to be in contact with the bed surface and place your top hand on the bed
- Tighten your abdominal muscles
- Gently swing your lower legs off the edge of the bed; at the same time, push your upper trunk into an erect position using both your bottom elbow and top hand
- Once in a seated position, lean forward slightly and use your hands to lift your weight off the bed, allowing your feet to contact the floor

Sleeping on Your Back

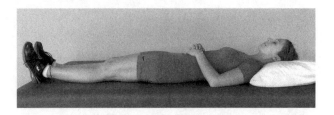

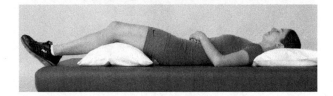

- When lying on your back, position yourself so that your head is supported by the pillow without being propped up too far
- Avoid having your arms over your head for extended periods; leaving them at your side, or across your abdomen, is preferred
- Have your knees slightly bent with a pillow under your knees for enhanced support
- Avoid crossing one leg over the other while sleeping

Sleeping on Your Side

B6

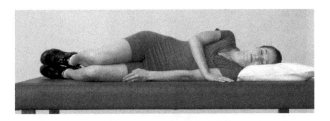

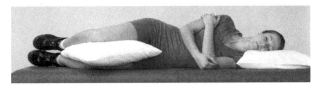

- When lying on your side, be sure that the pillow is not doubled or propped up too far

- Your head and neck should be in line with the rest of your body in this position

- Placing a pillow between your knees will help to keep your pelvis and lower spine in a neutral position

- Hand/arm positions are variable; avoid lying with one arm beneath any part of your body or head while in this position

B7 Standing in a Working Position

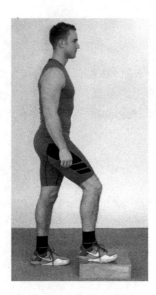

- Position yourself close to the table or other work surface you are facing

- Avoid leaning forward or straining your neck forward

- Consider having one knee slightly bent by resting it on a thick book or block of wood; if you're in front of a sink, open the cabinet beneath the sink and rest your foot on the cabinet shelf; in both scenarios, alternate your feet in this position

- Keep your abdominal muscles engaged to keep your lower back supported

- Take frequent breaks to stand up tall and stretch if you spend more than five minutes at this task

Sitting at the Computer   B8

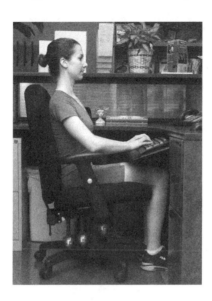

- Keep your feet flat on the floor and your legs uncrossed
- Using a low stool or pivoting footrest can help bring your hips into a 90-degree angle to your spine, which can help alleviate fatigue
- Your knees should be bent to 90-degree angles as you work, but repositioning them frequently can help avoid achiness of the legs and calves
- Position yourself so that you can sit with your back supported by the back of the chair
- Using pillows or lumbar supports can make it easier to feel support from the back of the chair
- Avoid leaning forward as you sit
- Always maintain a small hollow in your lower back and engage your abdominal muscles

Adjusting Your Monitor

- Your eye level should be within the top third of the monitor screen when you're seated upright

- The monitor should be positioned approximately twenty inches from your eyes, but feel free to adjust it to avoid having to squint or incline your head forward to improve focus

- Avoid glare on your monitor by making sure it's as close to perpendicular (a 90-degree angle) to the light source as possible; this may mean adjusting the orientation of the monitor to the windows in your workstation

- If you find yourself leaning toward the screen to read it, you may need to adjust the position of the monitor or use reading glasses or bifocals to read comfortably

Adjusting Your Keyboard

- Use the armrests of your chair to support your forearms so that you don't have to hold the weight of your arms with your shoulder and neck muscles

- Your wrists should be in a neutral position (not bent forward or cocked backward) as you type

- You may benefit from using gel pads or wrist rests to support your wrists as you type or use your mouse

- Keep the keyboard flat or very slightly tilted upward in the back for optimal positioning

- While seated, you should be able to rest your fingers on the keyboard with your elbows bent to a 90-degree angle, with your wrists in a neutral or flat position

Reaching Into a Low Drawer   B10

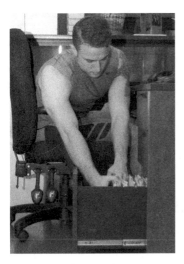
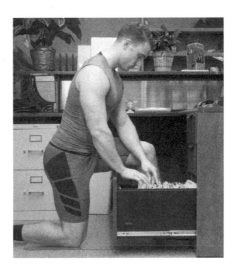

Incorrect   *Correct*

One of the day-to-day stresses in the low back is repetitive bending and twisting while sitting at your desk. Such movement may seem negligible, but it can significantly impact your recovery. Although it takes a bit more effort to get out of your chair to reach into lower desk drawers, your back will thank you. Here's how to do it correctly:

- Avoid twisting and bending
- Get up out of your chair, and face the drawer
- Drop to one knee to lower your center of gravity
- Tighten your abdominal muscles to support your spine
- Open the drawer or file cabinet without twisting

B11

Using the Telephone

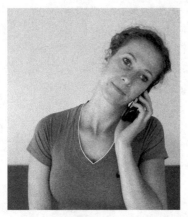
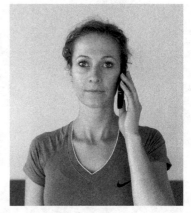

Incorrect   *Correct*

Many of us spend considerable time on the phone. Unfortunately, too many people end up holding their phone as shown above. This is stressful on the neck and can contribute to chronic neck pain if done on a regular basis. When speaking on the phone, follow these general rules:

- Avoid cradling the phone between your ear and shoulder while tipping your neck to the side
- Hold your phone to your ear with your hand
- Consider using a headset or Bluetooth device to minimize use of your hands
- If standing and speaking on the phone for more than a few minutes, prop one foot up on a stool or elevated surface, and bear weight equally through your legs and feet

Reading While Sitting

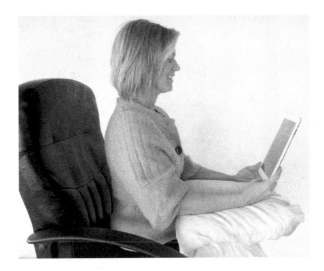

Reading requires that you stay in one position for an extended period of time. As long as this is done properly, it should not place undue strain on your neck and upper back. Here are some suggestions to help minimize the stress on your body while you read:

- Consider using pillows to help support both your arms and the book, magazine, or tablet you're reading to minimize strain on your neck and shoulders

- Avoid sitting to the side or with your legs tucked under you while reading

- Keep your feet supported on the floor or on a low footstool

- Take frequent breaks and walk around

B13 Washing Machine - Front Loading

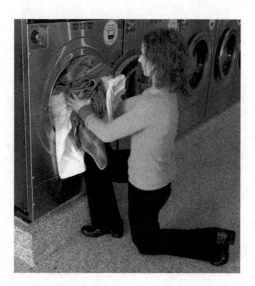

- Tighten your abdominal muscles as you face the washer
- Lower yourself onto one knee with the other knee forward while supporting your trunk with your arms
- Open the washer door
- Position yourself as close to the washer as possible
- Take small handfuls of clothes out of the washer and bring them close to your stomach
- Continue to keep your abdominal muscles tight
- Step away from the washer while holding the clothes close to your belly button before moving them to the dryer or a basket

Washing Machine- Top Loading   B14

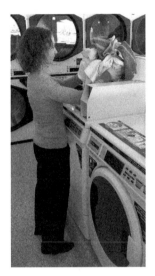
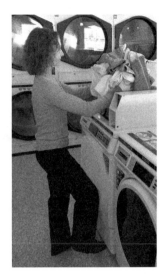

Incorrect   *Correct*

Doing laundry can be quite stressful on the back and neck. Not only do you have to do a lot of bending and reaching, but the added weight and bulk of your laundry can significantly increase the level of stress on your body. Follow the guidelines below when using a top-loading washing machine to reduce your risk of injury:

- Get as close to the machine as possible with one foot slightly in front of the other
- Reach into the washer without twisting
- Tighten your abdominal muscles before you lift
- Take small handfuls of clothes out of the washer and bring them close to your stomach
- Step away from the washer while holding the clothes close to your belly button before moving them to the dryer or a basket

B15 Reaching into the Refrigerator

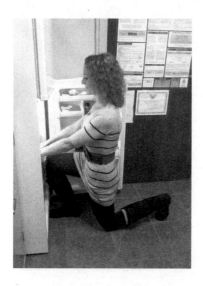 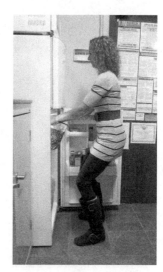

- Slide the object toward you as close to the edge of the shelf as possible; this may require some repositioning of surrounding objects

- Bring your body as close to the shelf as possible

- If possible, keep your elbows bent and close to your body before you lift something off the shelf

- As you prepare to lift, tighten your abdominal muscles and slightly bend your knees, maintaining your trunk in an erect posture

- As you hold the object, make sure you are comfortable with its weight before lifting it off the shelf

- As you bring the object off the shelf, keep your elbows bent and close to your body; bend your knees slightly and hold the object as close to your body as possible

- Once the object is secure, turn while holding it directly in front of you

Low Shelf Squat

B16

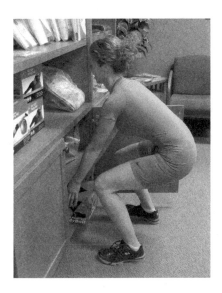

- Tighten your abdominal muscles to help support your pelvis
- Squat down, keeping your trunk erect; avoid bending at the waist
- Slide the object toward you as close to the edge of the shelf as possible; this may require some repositioning of surrounding objects
- Bring your body as close to the shelf as possible
- As you bring the object off the shelf, keep your elbows bent and close to your body
- Once the object is secure, tighten your abdominal muscles and straighten your legs, keeping the object as close to your center of gravity (your belly button) as possible
- Turn to walk away, keeping the object directly in front of you
- Avoid twisting with the object outside your center of gravity

Low Shelf Half Kneel

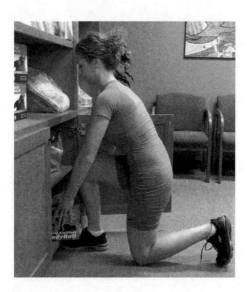

- Tighten your abdominal muscles, keeping your pelvis supported
- Lower your body to position yourself in a half- kneeling posture; get your trunk as close to the shelf or drawer as possible
- Slide the object toward you as close to the edge of the shelf as possible; this may require some repositioning of surrounding objects
- If possible, keep your elbows bent and close to your body before lifting something off the shelf
- As you bring the object off the shelf, keep your elbows bent and close to your body
- Once the object is secure, tighten your abdominal muscles and straighten your legs, keeping the object as close to your center of gravity (your belly button) as possible
- Turn to walk away, keeping the object directly in front of you
- Avoid twisting with the object outside your center of gravity

Placing Objects on a High Shelf   B18

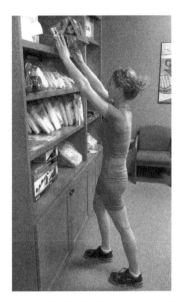

Lifting objects onto or off of a high surface, such as on top of a refrigerator or on the top shelf of a cabinet, introduces additional stresses on both the neck and low back. In order to minimize the risk of injury, follow these guidelines:

- Stand with feet hip width apart or slightly wider, holding object at your belly button
- Place one foot as close to the shelf as possible
- Perform a pelvic tilt by pulling your belly button toward your spine to engage your abdominal muscles
- Bend your knees slightly
- Shift weight forward onto front foot as you straighten your knees
- Use arms to lift object from your belly button to the shelf; shift your weight forward as you slide it onto the shelf
- Reverse these steps to remove an object from a high shelf

Squat Lifting

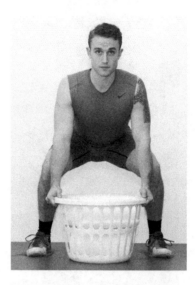

- Stand with your feet hip-width apart, facing the object to be lifted
- Perform a pelvic tilt by pulling your belly button toward your spine to engage your abdominal muscles
- Squat down as close to the object as possible to lower your center of gravity
- Before you lift the item, bring it as close to you as possible (by sliding it along the floor if you can)
- Tighten your abdominal muscles again
- Lift the object and bring it close to your belly button
- Keep your spine straight
- Stand erect by straightening your knees, using your legs and gluteal muscles to lift the object

Half-Kneel Lifting

B20

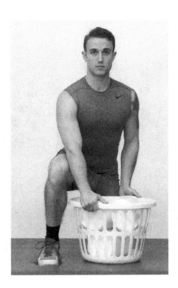

- Stand with your feet hip-width apart, facing the object to be lifted
- Perform a pelvic tilt by pulling your belly button toward your spine to engage your abdominal muscles
- Lower one knee toward the floor to lower your center of gravity
- Move as close to the object as possible
- Before you lift the item, bring it as close to you as possible (by sliding it along the floor if you can)
- Tighten your abdominal muscles again
- Lift the object and bring it close to your belly button
- Keep your spine straight
- Stand erect by straightening your knees, using your legs and gluteal muscles to lift the object

B21
Bending to Lift

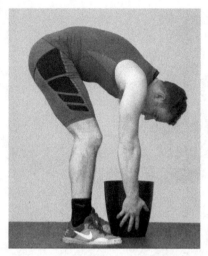
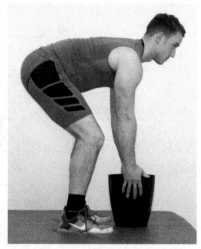

Incorrect   *Correct*

- Bending is the least optimal way to lift, but it can be performed if other types of lifting are not feasible
- Keep your back and neck in line (do not allow your back to round out)
- Bend your knees as much as possible
- Lower your buttocks as low as possible
- When you are as close to the object as you can get, tighten your abdominal muscles
- Very carefully, lift the object, bringing it as close to your belly button as possible

Golfer's Lift

B22

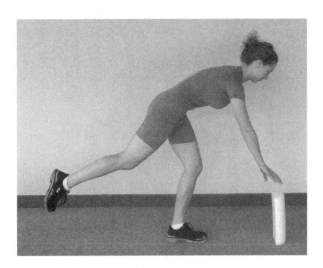

- Stand slightly behind the object you wish to pick up (this works best for smaller and/or lighter objects)

- Keep your front leg planted and your knee slightly bent

- Begin to bend forward at the waist, flexing the hip of the front leg but keeping the spine straight as you lift the back leg off the floor to stabilize yourself, keeping the back knee as straight as possible; your back foot should come one to two feet off the floor, with the motion to reach toward the floor coming mainly from your hips

- Return to standing position by bringing your back leg back down to the floor, while at the same time extending your hips until you're in an upright position

Vacuuming

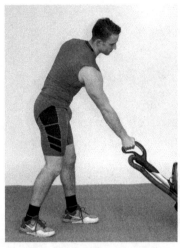 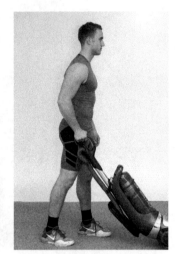

Incorrect   *Correct*

The repetitive nature of vacuuming can lead to re-injury fairly quickly. Here are a few tips to minimize the stress on your back from vacuuming:

- Keep your abdominal muscles firm before attempting to move the vacuum
- Position yourself so that you are grabbing the end of the handle
- The handle should be at the level of your belly button
- Bend your knees slightly
- Avoid bending or twisting your back
- Place one foot behind the other and slightly off to the side
- Shift your body weight back and forth from foot to foot to move the vacuum forward and back
- When you are turning the vacuum, let the vacuum head roll as you move your body around to stay behind the handle
- Never attempt to lift the vacuum by the handle

Sweeping and Raking

B24

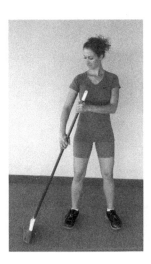

- The most important things to keep in mind while sweeping or raking are to keep your spine neutral and to avoid twisting

- Stand with the broom or rake in front of you with the head of it perpendicular to your body, starting with it close to your right foot

- Keeping the broom or rake close to your body, gently reach out about one foot in front of your right foot, then pull it toward your left foot

- Take a step to the left and repeat these steps

B25

Shoveling

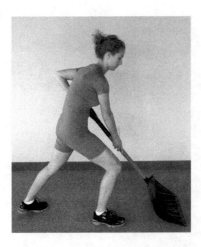
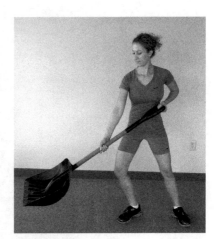

- Place yourself perpendicular to the snow you are going to shovel

- Lunging slightly forward with your front knee bent, slightly bend at the waist to ensure that your spine stays neutral; reach out slightly (no more than twelve inches) to scoop snow into the shovel (keeping the load light to medium)

- Get your body and center of gravity as close to the load as possible before lifting

- Pivoting on your feet and avoiding any twist in your spine, step away with your back leg, shifting your weight onto your rear leg while bending at the knee

- Once your hips are pivoted all the way around using your core muscles and a weight shift from the back to the front leg, push the shovel away from your body to unload the snow

- Pivot on your feet back to the starting position to scoop the next shovelful; move your feet and side step when necessary

Shopping

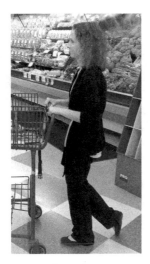 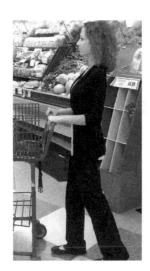

Incorrect   *Correct*

- While pushing a shopping cart, stand tall as opposed to leaning into the cart and bending at the waist

- Keep your abdominal muscles firm as you prepare to push

- Drive the cart forward with your legs, bending at the knees to propel it forward

B27

Getting into a Vehicle

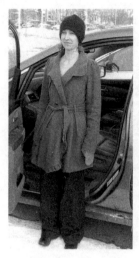 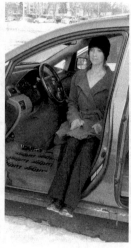 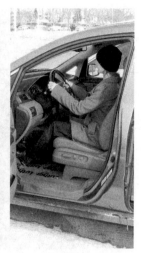

This step-by-step process is the best way to ensure that you enter a vehicle from the driver's side with minimal stress and strain on your spine:

- Position yourself so that your back faces the middle of the front seat

- Slowly bend at the knees and hips, keeping your spine straight

- Use your hands to feel the surface of the seat and to help lower yourself into a seated position

- You may need to look downward or bend your head forward to avoid hitting it on the roof of the vehicle

- Once you are seated, perform a pelvic tilt by pulling your belly button toward your spine to engage your abdominal muscles

- Gently pivot on your buttocks, swinging both legs together into the car and toward the pedals

- Keep your spine from twisting, and sit erect as you fasten your seat belt

Getting out of a Vehicle

B28

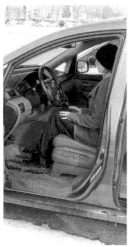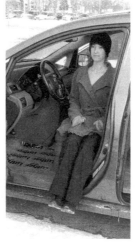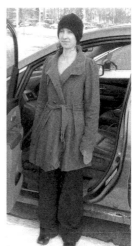

This step-by-step process is the best way to ensure that you exit a vehicle from the driver's side with minimal stress and strain on your spine:

- Bend your knees so that your feet are together
- Perform a pelvic tilt by pulling your belly button toward your spine to engage your abdominal muscles
- Use your hands to push down on the seat to raise your buttocks slightly, enabling your hips to turn toward the door while moving your feet and knees as a unit
- Make small positional shifts with your knees together until you face the door with your feet outside the vehicle and on the ground
- Use your hands to push off the seat as you move your buttocks toward the edge of the car's front seat
- Tighten your abdominal muscles
- Keeping your spine in line, stand up, bending your head slightly to avoid the roof of the vehicle

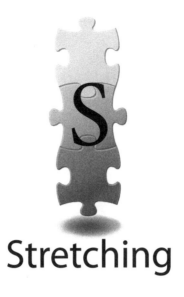

Stretching

The DMR Method includes a unique system of stretching called Integrated Progressive Stretching and Flexibility techniques. This system is designed to help patients safely and effectively stretch through all three phases of the DMR Method.

Only perform the stretches given to you by your DMR Method provider and make sure to follow the five rules of stretching:

- Warm up before stretching; walk in place for a couple minutes to warm your body and slightly raise your heart rate (if your condition prevents you from safely warming up, follow the instructions of your provider on proper initial stretching techniques)

- Never stretch your muscles too aggressively; only stretch to the point where you can feel a mild pull on the muscle; stretching should not be painful

- Never bounce while stretching

- Maintain proper positioning

- Hold each stretch for forty-five to sixty seconds

IMPORTANT! Be sure to keep all stretched pain-free! If you feel pain, stop the stretch and talk to your clinician about adapting the stretch for your comfort.

SC1

Upper Trapezius

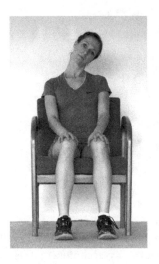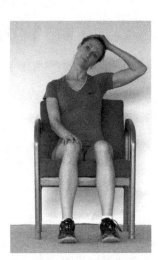

- Sit with good posture
- Keeping your nose pointing straight ahead, tilt your head to bring one ear straight down toward your shoulder until you feel a good stretch
- If instructed to do so, place your hand (from the side you're leaning toward) on top of your head and add extra pulling pressure
- Hold for forty-five to sixty seconds
- Gently return to neutral position, then repeat the stretch on the other side
- Complete one repetition on each side
- Repeat two to three times per day

Levator

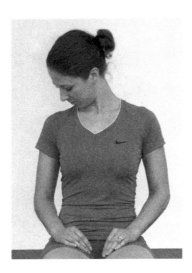

- Sit with good posture
- Turn your head 45 degrees, then bring your nose down toward the same armpit until you feel a stretch on the back side of your neck on the opposite side
- If instructed to do so, bring your hand (from the side you're leaning toward) to the back of your head and add extra pull to bring your nose closer to your armpit
- Hold for forty-five to sixty seconds
- Gently return to neutral position, then repeat the stretch on the other side
- Complete one repetition on each side
- Repeat two to three times per day

SC3

Cervical Extension

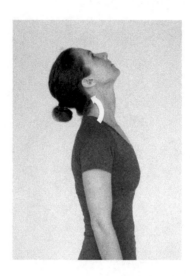

- From a neutral seated or standing position, slowly extend your neck backward in an arc until you feel a gentle stretch in the front of your neck

- Hold for forty-five to sixty seconds

- Complete one repetition

- Repeat two to three times per day

- Note: stop this stretch immediately if you experience any dizziness

Scalenes

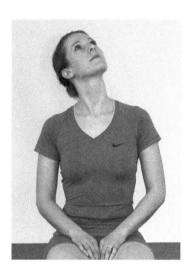

- Sit with good posture
- Tip your ear toward your shoulder, then rotate your chin and nose up in the opposite direction toward the ceiling as far as is comfortable
- The goal is to stretch the front side of your neck without pinching on the back side of your neck
- Gently return to the neutral position, then repeat the same or alternative stretch on the other side
- Each side of the neck may be done in a different way depending on your symptoms
- Hold for forty-five to sixty seconds
- Complete one repetition on each side of the neck
- Repeat two to three times per day

Shoulder Rolls

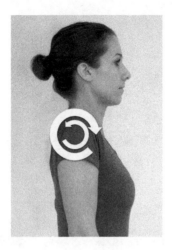

- Stand with your arms at your side
- Slowly raise your shoulders up toward your ears
- Rotate your shoulders back while squeezing your shoulder blades together
- Continue the rotation slowly toward the floor and then forward so that your shoulder blades stretch apart
- Return to the starting position
- Repeat five times, then do the same stretch in the opposite direction five times
- Repeat two to three times per day

Pectoralis

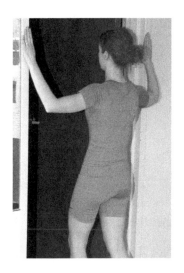 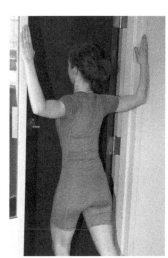

- Stand in a doorframe
- Place your forearms flush on the doorjambs at a 90-degree angle to your shoulder and elbows
- Standing tall and keeping your head in line with your body, take a small step forward with one foot until you feel a stretch on the front of your chest and shoulders
- Hold for forty-five to sixty seconds
- Return to the starting position then move your arms up the doorframe two to three inches; repeat the stretch again
- Complete each stretch one time
- Repeat two to three times per day

Rhomboid Gas Pedal

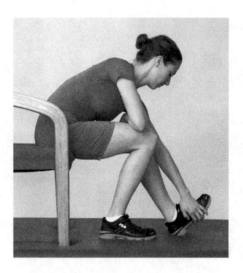

- Sit forward on the edge of a chair
- Place one foot forward, putting the heel on the ground with your toes slightly up in the air with your other knee bent at 90 degrees
- Lean forward, bracing your forearm or chest on your thighs then grab the outside of the foot on the same side with your thumb pointed upwards (for a deeper stretch, reach around to the inside of the foot if you can comfortably do so as pictured above)
- Without moving your body, keep holding your foot while pushing it toward the ground like you're pushing on a gas pedal
- Hold for forty-five to sixty seconds
- Repeat the stretch on the other side with the other foot
- Complete one repetition on each side
- Repeat two to three times per day

Rhomboid Doorway

SC8

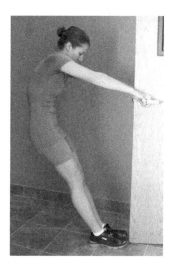

- Stand next to an open sturdy door

- Grab the handle on both sides of the door simultaneously

- Place your feet close to the door. Keeping your legs and arms straight, start to lean back (you can allow your upper back to round slightly while tucking your chin to your chest to increase the stretch). Continue to lean back until you feel a stretch between your shoulder blades.

- Hold for forty-five to sixty seconds

- Complete one repetition

- Repeat two to three times per day

Rhomboid Sitting

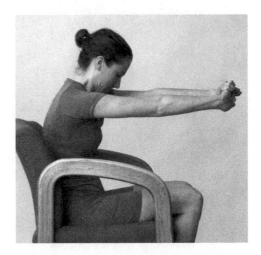

- Sit with good posture
- Clasp hands in front of you at shoulder level
- Reach forward, slightly rounding your shoulders and tucking your chin down until you feel a stretch between your shoulder blades
- Hold for forty-five to sixty seconds
- Taking a deep breath and holding it may increase the stretch
- Complete one repetition
- Repeat two to three times per day

Thoracic Shimmies

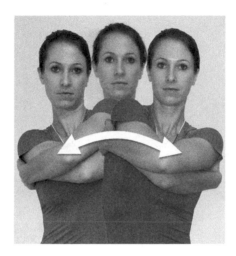

- From a neutral seated or standing position, cross your arms across your chest
- Slightly lean from side to side at a rate of about one repetition per second
- Imagine you are side-bending around an axis in the middle of your back
- Continue for forty-five to sixty seconds
- Repeat two to three times per day

Prayer Stretch

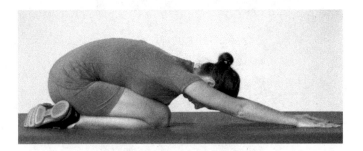

- Start on your hands and knees
- Keeping your hands where they are, slowly sit back onto your heels
- Gently tuck your head down between your elbows until you feel a stretch at the back of your shoulders or in your back
- Hold for forty-five to sixty seconds
- Complete one repetition
- Repeat two to three times per day

Quadratus Lumborum

SC12

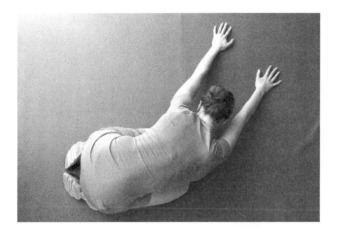

- Start in the prayer position
- Move your left hand one to two feet toward the left
- Put your right hand beside your left hand to curve your spine into a slight C with your hips moving toward your hands
- Hold for forty-five to sixty seconds
- Relax and repeat on the other side
- Complete one repetition on each side
- Repeat two to three times per day

Cat / Camel Stretch

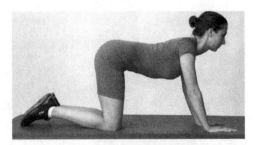

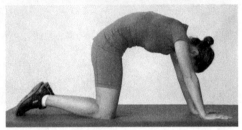

- Start on your hands and knees
- Sink your spine down toward the floor, lifting your head up slightly to make a U shape with your body
- Hold ten seconds
- Reverse the movement and lift your spine up toward the ceiling, tucking your chin down like an angry cat, making an upside down U with your body
- Hold ten seconds
- Continue to move back and forth to each position until you have completed five repetitions in each position
- Repeat two to three times per day

Single-Knee to Chest

SL1

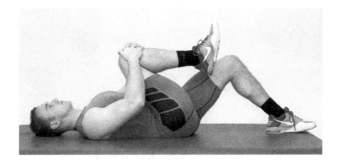

- Lie on your back on the floor (or on your bed if it's too painful for you to perform this stretch on the floor)
- Gently bring one knee to your chest, pulling until you feel a gentle stretch (your hands can either be on top of or behind your knee)
- Hold for forty-five to sixty seconds
- Slowly return your foot to the floor
- Repeat on the other side
- Complete one repetition on each side
- Repeat two to three times per day

Double-Knee to Chest

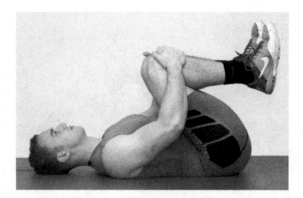

- Lie on your back on the floor (or on your bed if it's too painful for you to perform this stretch on the floor)
- Pull your knees into your chest one at a time until you feel a gentle stretch (your hands can either be on top of or behind your knees)
- Hold for forty-five to sixty seconds
- Gently return your feet to the floor
- Complete one repetition
- Repeat two to three times per day

Pelvic Rolls

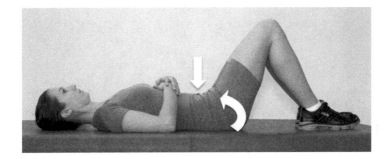

- Lie on your back on the floor (or on your bed if it's too painful for you to perform this stretch on the floor)
- Tighten your abdominal muscles by drawing your belly button toward your spine
- Rotate your pelvis backward so that your low back pushes into the floor
- Hold this position forty-five to sixty seconds while continuing to breathe
- Allow your muscles to relax, then rotate your pelvis forward back to the starting position
- Complete three repetitions
- Repeat two to three times per day

SL4

Trunk Rotation

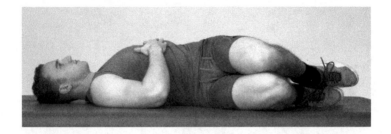

- Lie on your back on the floor (or on your bed if it's too painful for you to perform this stretch on the floor) with your knees bent up and your feet together flat on the surface
- Keeping your shoulders down, gently drop your knees toward the floor, allowing your feet to rotate off the floor until you feel a gentle stretch
- To increase the stretch (if instructed to do so by your provider), straighten your top leg while keeping the hip flexed
- Hold for forty-five to sixty seconds
- Gently bring your knees back to the center, then rotate to the opposite side and hold for forty-five to sixty seconds
- Complete one repetition to each side
- Repeat two to three times per day

Piriformis on Mat

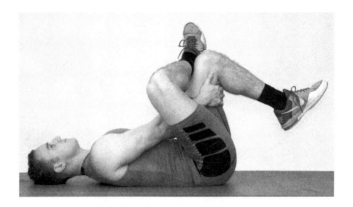

- Lie on your back on the floor (or on your bed if it's too painful for you to perform this stretch on the floor) with your knees bent and your feet flat on the surface

- Cross one leg over the other so that your ankle rests on your opposite knee

- If you feel a stretch in this position, stop there and hold the stretch for forty-five to sixty seconds; if no stretch is felt, begin to pull the opposite leg toward your chest until you feel a gentle stretch

- Hold for forty-five to sixty seconds

- Gently return to neutral position, then repeat the stretch on the other side, holding it for forty-five to sixty seconds

- Complete one repetition on each side

- Repeat two to three times per day

Seated Piriformis

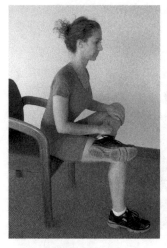
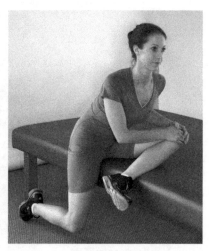

Technique 1   *Technique 2*

- Sit with good posture in a chair or on the edge of a bed or bench, positioning yourself as shown above
- Keep your spine in a neutral position (as if a rod is in your spine)
- Lean forward from the hips until you feel a stretch in the leg that is crossed
- Hold for forty-five to sixty seconds
- Repeat the stretch with the other leg, holding it for forty-five to sixty seconds
- Complete one repetition on each side
- Repeat two to three times per day

Hamstring Supine

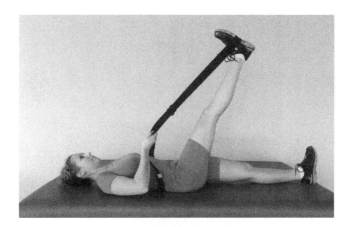

- Lie on your back on the floor (or on your bed if it's too painful for you to perform this stretch on the floor) with both knees bent and your feet flat on the surface

- Place a towel or belt around one foot (keeping it in the arch of the foot) and extend your leg until your knee is straight

- Begin to pull the strap toward your head, raising your leg up until you feel a stretch in the back of the leg; to increase the stretch you can straighten the opposite knee

- Hold for forty-five to sixty seconds

- Return to the starting position, then repeat the stretch on the other leg for forty-five to sixty seconds

- Repeat two to three times per day

SL8

Hamstring Seated

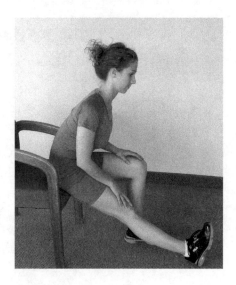

- Sit on the edge of a chair with good posture
- Stretch one leg out in front of you with the heel on the floor and your foot relaxed; the other knee should be bent to 90 degrees with your foot flat on the floor
- Keeping your spine straight, lean forward (as if you are hinging forward from the hips) until you feel a gentle stretch in the back of the straight leg
- Hold for forty-five to sixty seconds
- Repeat the stretch with the other leg for forty-five to sixty seconds
- Complete one repetition on each side
- Repeat two to three times per day

Hamstring Wall

SL9

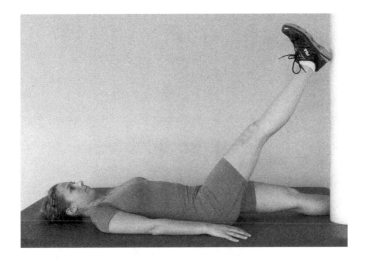

- Lie in a doorway or position yourself near a wall so that one leg can go up the wall and the other leg can extend straight out in front of you
- Place your foot on the wall with your heel contacting the wall and the foot relaxed
- Move closer to the wall with your body until you feel a comfortable stretch in the back of your leg, making sure your knee is totally straight
- Hold for forty-five to sixty seconds
- Bring that leg down and move to the other side of the doorframe or wall to repeat the stretch with the other leg
- Complete one repetition on each leg
- Repeat two to three times per day

Quadriceps Standing

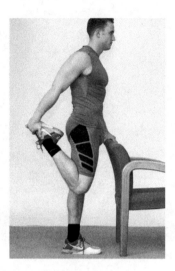

- Stand up straight with good posture
- Hold onto a chair or counter to maintain your balance
- Raise one heel toward your buttock
- Grasp your ankle and pull heel toward your buttock until you feel a stretch on the front of the thigh
- Make sure to keep the knee of the stretched leg pointing toward the floor
- Hold for forty-five to sixty seconds
- Put that foot back on the floor and repeat the stretch on the other side for forty-five to sixty seconds
- Complete one repetition on each side
- Repeat two to three times per day

Quadriceps Towel Stretch   SL11

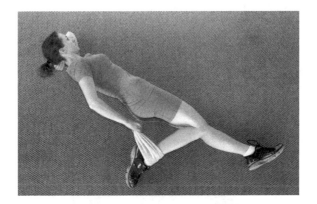

- Lie on your side on the floor or in bed
- Loop a towel or belt around the ankle of your top leg
- Keeping your body in a straight line (avoid arching your back), pull your ankle toward your buttock until you feel a stretch in the front of the thigh
- Hold for forty-five to sixty seconds
- Roll to your other side and repeat on the opposite leg for forty-five to sixty seconds
- Complete one repetition on each side
- Repeat two to three times per day

SL12

Hip Flexor Lunge - High

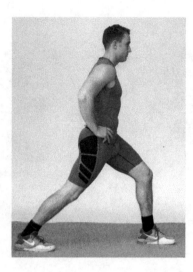

- Stand up straight with your toes pointed forward on both feet
- Take one step forward into a lunge position, bringing the front leg two feet in front of the back leg
- Perform a pelvic tilt by pulling your belly button toward your spine to engage your abdominal muscles
- Bend the front knee slightly (avoid leaning forward from the hips) until a stretch is felt in the straight leg
- Hold for forty-five to sixty seconds
- Return to the starting position and switch to the opposite leg, repeating the stretch forty-five to sixty seconds
- Complete one repetition on each side
- Repeat two to three times per day

Hip Flexor Lunge - Chair   SL13

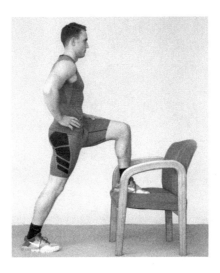

- Standing straight with good posture, place one leg up on a chair, making sure that your toes on both feet point straight ahead
- Keeping your trunk over your pelvis, perform a pelvic tilt by pulling your belly button toward your spine to engage your abdominal muscles
- Keeping your back leg straight, bend the forward knee (avoid leaning forward from the hips), moving your body weight onto the front foot until a stretch is felt in the straight leg
- Hold for forty-five to sixty seconds
- Bring that foot down to the floor, switch to the opposite leg and repeat the stretch for forty-five to sixty seconds
- Complete one repetition on each side
- Repeat two to three times per day

SL14

Hip Flexor- Low

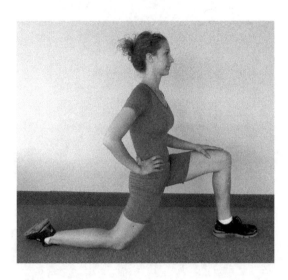

- Kneel down on one knee with the opposite leg forward in a lunge position, with knees shoulder-width apart and your back knee and front foot pointing straight ahead

- Keep your back straight and your trunk over your pelvis; do not lean forward

- Bend the forward knee until a stretch is felt in the front of the back leg near the front of the groin or thigh

- Make sure your front knee is not in front of your toes. If you are unable to do this, reset your position, placing your front foot further forward

- Hold for forty-five to sixty seconds

- Return to the starting position, switch to the opposite leg and repeat the stretch for forty-five to sixty seconds

- Complete one repetition on each side

- Repeat two to three times per day

Hip Flexor-Leg Hang

SL15

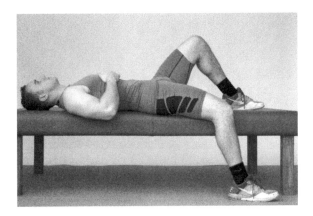

- Lie on your back toward the edge of a bed or bench with your knees bent and your feet flat on the surface
- Let your leg hang off the edge of the bed or bench, leaving the other knee bent
- Allow gravity to pull your leg toward the floor
- Hold for forty-five to sixty seconds
- Return to the starting position, then turn your body around and repeat the stretch with the other leg for forty-five to sixty seconds
- Complete one repetition on each side
- Repeat two to three times per day

SL16

Hip Adductor-Seated

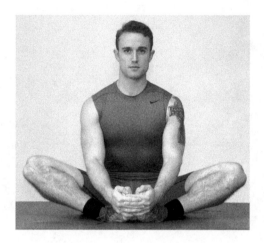

- Sit on the floor with your back against a wall
- Grasp your feet with your hands and press the soles of your feet together
- Sitting up tall, begin to pull your feet toward your pelvis as far as you comfortably can, then gently allow your knees to drop toward the floor until you feel a stretch on the inside portion of your thighs
- Hold for forty-five to sixty seconds
- Complete one repetition
- Repeat two to three times per day

Gastrocnemius and Soleus   SL17

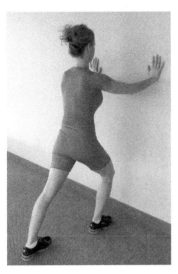 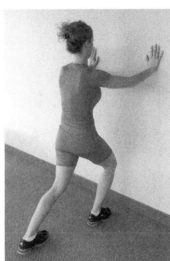

- Stand facing a wall with one foot positioned in front of the other; your back foot should be about two feet away from the wall and your front foot should be a few inches from the wall. Ensure that both feet are pointing straight forward
- Keep your back knee straight and both feet flat on the floor
- Start to bend the front knee, shifting weight more onto that foot until you feel a stretch in the calf area of the back leg
- Hold for forty-five to sixty seconds
- Next, bend the back knee about 15 degrees to change the stretch; you should now feel the stretch more in the ankle
- Hold for forty-five to sixty seconds
- Switch legs and repeat both stretches on the other leg
- Complete one repetition of both stretches on each leg
- Repeat two to three times per day

Femoral Nerve Flossing

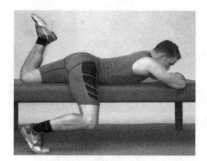 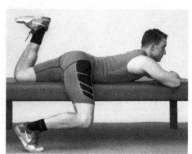

- Lay face down with your pain-free leg hanging off the bench or bed
- Bend up the opposite leg and bring your heel toward your buttock (you can use a towel or strap to help keep your knee bent)
- As your heel approaches your buttock, look down to bring your chin toward your chest
- Hold for five seconds
- Next, point your toes toward the bench or bed and lift your head to look upwards
- Hold for five seconds
- Repeat this pattern for one minute
- Repeat three times per day

Sciatic Nerve Flossing   `SL19`

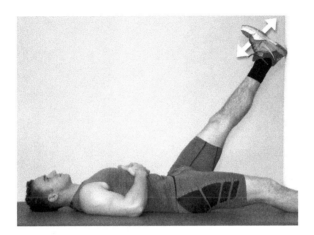

- Lie on your back with your legs straight
- Begin to raise the leg with symptoms into the air until you feel a pull either in your back or down your leg
- Bring the leg down from that position two inches until you no longer feel any discomfort in your back or leg; rest the leg on a pillow, doorframe, or piece of furniture
- Slowly pull your toes toward your nose on the symptomatic leg, until the pull in your back or leg returns
- Hold for five seconds
- Point your toes toward the wall until the pull goes away; hold for five seconds
- Repeat this pattern for one minute
- Complete one repetition on the painful leg
- Repeat two to three times per day
- To increase the flossing effect, bring your head up when your toes are pointed toward the wall and lay your head down when your toes are pointed toward your head

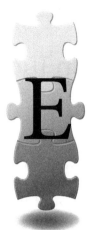

Stabilizing Exercises

The DMR Method is designed to strengthen and stabilize your body by providing you with exercises tailored to your personal needs. Your provider will introduce basic conditioning exercises when appropriate and then progress to advanced stabilization exercises as you move through the three phases of recovery. Be patient and only perform the exercises given to you by your provider. In addition to these strengthening and stabilization exercises, you will be given recommendations for appropriate aerobic exercise that will help improve your endurance and cardiovascular health.

> **IMPORTANT!** *Be sure to keep all exercises pain-free! If you feel pain, stop the exercise and talk to your clinician about adapting the exercise for your comfort.*

Aerobic Exercise

As part of the DMR Method program, light aerobic exercise is encouraged as soon as you reach the repair phase of recovery. The main benefits of aerobic exercise are improving endurance and cardiovascular health. Aerobic exercise should be performed three to five days per week for a minimum of twenty minutes per day. Depending on your specific condition, your providers will recommend optimal forms of aerobic exercise. Options include:

Walking	Treadmill	Light jogging
Swimming	Stationary bike	Recumbent bike
Elliptical machine	Stair-climber	Rowing machine

Only do the aerobic exercises approved by your DMR Method provider.

Chin Tucks

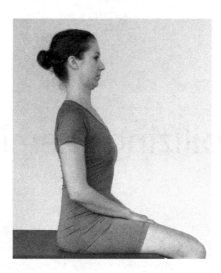

- Sit with good posture
- Slowly move your chin straight back one to two inches until your ears are in line with your shoulders (if needed, you can place your hand on your chin to guide the backward movement)
- Keep this movement pain free (if you feel pain or an uncomfortable stretch at the base of the skull, decrease the range of movement until you are pain free)
- Hold for five seconds, then return to the starting position
- Complete ten repetitions
- Repeat five times per day

Scapular Retraction

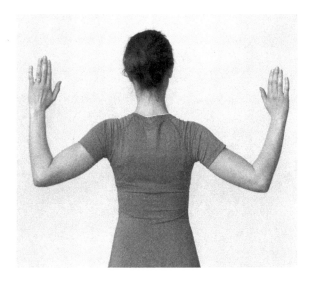

- Sit or stand with good posture
- Bring your arms up to 90 degrees at your shoulders and elbows (if this is uncomfortable, this exercise can be performed with your arms resting at your sides)
- Squeeze your shoulder blades down and together in a "V" motion
- Keep the movement pain free
- Hold for five seconds, then return to the starting position
- Complete ten repetitions
- Repeat five times per day

EC3 # Cervical Isometric Flexion

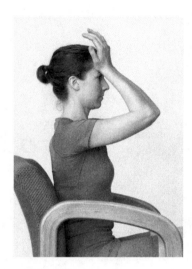

- Sit with good posture
- Place the heels of both hands on your forehead, keeping your head in a neutral position (if this is uncomfortable ,you can bring your arms down and use your fingertips)
- Gently push your forehead into your hands, pushing as hard as you comfortably can while applying an equivalent amount of counter-pressure with your hands to keep your head in a neutral position
- Keep the exercise pain free
- Hold for five seconds, then rest
- Complete ten repetitions
- Perform once per day

Cervical Side Flexion

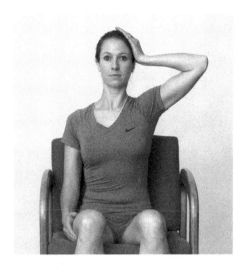

- Sit with good posture with your head in a neutral position
- Place the heel of one hand on the side of your head above your ear, keeping your head in a neutral position (f this position is painful for your arm or causes a tingling sensation, bring your arm down slightly and use your fingertips instead, but be sure that your head does not tip to the side)
- Gently push your head into your hand as hard as you comfortably can while applying an equivalent amount of counter-pressure with your hand to keep your head in a neutral position
- Keep the exercise pain free
- Hold for five seconds, then rest
- Complete ten repetitions
- Repeat the exercise on the other side with your other hand
- Perform once per day

Cervical Isometric Extension

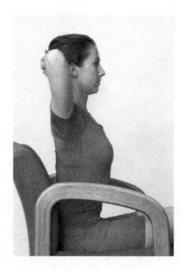

- Sit with good posture with your head in a neutral position
- Place both hands on the back of your head and lace your fingers together (if this exercise is painful for your arms, you can perform it lying on the floor or in bed and pushing your head into the floor or bed instead of into your hands)
- Gently push your head into your hands as hard as you comfortably can while applying an equivalent amount of counter-pressure with your hands to keep your head in a neutral position
- Keep the exercise pain free
- Hold for five seconds then rest
- Complete ten repetitions
- Repeat two to three times per day

Cervical Isotonic Flexion

EC6

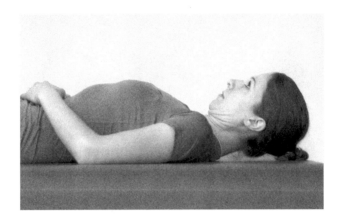

- Lie on your back on the floor or in bed
- Keep your shoulders and upper body relaxed and your shoulders drawn down toward your feet
- Gently tuck your chin into your chest, then curl your neck up like you're trying to touch your chin to your chest
- Keep the movement pain free
- Hold for three seconds
- Gently lower your head back down to the starting position, then release your chin tuck
- Complete ten repetitions
- Repeat in sets of ten repetitions with the goal of reaching thirty repetitions
- Stop immediately if your symptoms recur
- Repeat three to four times per week

EC7 Cervical Isotonic Lateral Flexion

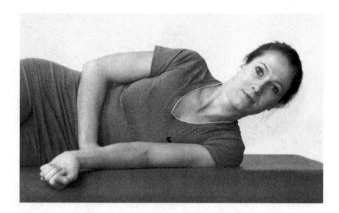

- Lie on your side on the floor or in a bed
- Keep your nose pointing straight to the horizon
- Bring your ear up toward your top shoulder, lifting your head off the floor or bed
- Keep the movement pain free
- Hold for three seconds
- Relax and bring your head back to the starting position
- Complete ten repetitions
- Repeat in sets of ten repetitions with the goal of reaching thirty repetitions
- Stop immediately if your symptoms recur
- Repeat three to four times per week
- Repeat on the other side by rolling over to the other shoulder

Cervical Isotonic Extension   EC8

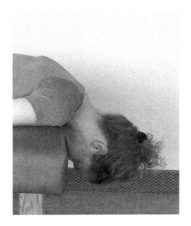 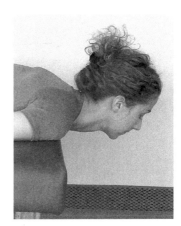

- Start by lying face down on the end of a bed with your shoulders on the edge of the bed and your head hanging off the end of the bed

- Curl your head back three inches like you're bringing the top of your head toward your feet, keeping your shoulders relaxed

- Keep the movement pain free

- Hold for three seconds, then gently lower your chin back down onto the end of the bed to the starting position

- Complete ten repetitions

- Repeat in sets of ten repetitions with the goal of reaching thirty repetitions

- Stop immediately if your symptoms recur

- Repeat three to four times per week

Rhomboid "T"

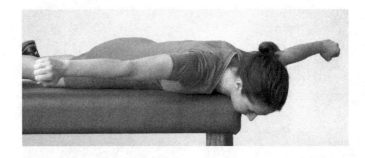

- Lie diagonally on a bed with both your arms hanging relaxed off the sides of the bed and your chin resting on the edge of the bed

- Gently squeeze your shoulder blades together and down toward your hips in a "V" position

- With your thumbs pointing down toward the floor, bring both your arms up toward the ceiling, keeping your elbows straight, until your arms are parallel to the floor and perpendicular to your trunk, forming the letter "T" with your body

- Hold for three seconds, then relax back into the starting position

- Complete ten repetitions

- Repeat in sets of ten repetitions with the goal of reaching thirty repetitions

- Stop immediately if your symptoms recur

- Repeat three to four times per week

- Once you reach your repetitions goal, your provider will show you how to perform this exercise with weights

Middle Trapezius "T"

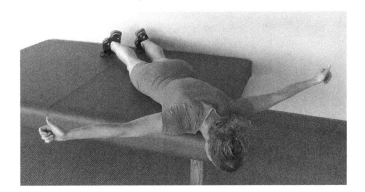

- Lie diagonally on a bed with both your arms hanging relaxed off the sides of the bed and your chin resting on the edge of the bed

- Gently squeeze your shoulder blades together and down toward your hips in a "V" position

- With your thumbs pointing up toward the ceiling, bring both your arms up toward the ceiling, keeping your elbows straight until your arms are parallel to the floor and perpendicular to your trunk, forming the letter "T" with your body

- Hold for three seconds, then relax back into the starting position

- Complete ten repetitions

- Repeat in sets of ten repetitions with the goal of reaching thirty repetitions

- Stop immediately if your symptoms recur

- Repeat three to four times per week

- Once you reach your repetitions goal, your provider will show you how to perform this exercise with weights

EC11

Lower Trapezius "Y"

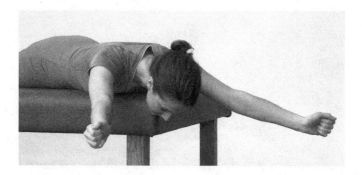

- Lie diagonally on a bed with both your arms hanging relaxed off the sides of the bed and your chin resting on the edge of the bed

- Gently squeeze your shoulder blades together and down toward your hips in a "V" position

- Lift your arms toward the ceiling with your arms forward in a "Y" shape with your thumbs pointing up toward the ceiling

- Hold for three seconds, then relax back into the starting position

- Complete ten repetitions

- Repeat in sets of ten repetitions with the goal of reaching thirty repetitions

- Stop immediately if your symptoms recur

- Repeat three to four times per week

- Once you reach your repetitions goal, your provider will show you how to perform this exercise with weights

Theraband Row

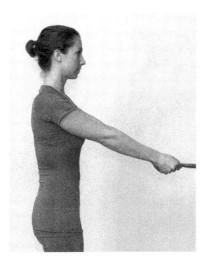 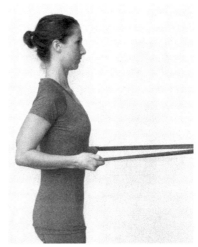

- Place a Theraband in a door with the knot at the level of your belly button
- Stand with good posture about two to three feet away from the doorjamb
- Grip the band in each hand
- Pull the band straight back toward your belly button, bending your elbows until your hands are at your sides
- While holding this position, squeeze your shoulder blades together five seconds
- Slowly return to the starting position
- As you get stronger, the motion of your arms and the squeezing of your shoulder blades can happen simultaneously
- Complete ten repetitions
- Perform two sets
- Repeat three to four times per week

EC13   Theraband Lat Pull-Down

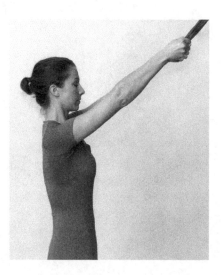
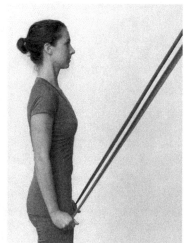

- Place a Theraband in the top of a doorjamb using a knot in the band to secure it in the shut door
- Stand with good posture facing the door so that your arms are straight out in front of you and about one inch away from the door with your elbows locked
- Pull your shoulder blades together and down toward your hips in a "V" position
- Keeping your arms straight, pull straight down until your hands are at your hips
- Hold five seconds
- Slowly return to the starting position
- As you get stronger, the motion of your arms and the squeezing of your shoulder blades can happen simultaneously
- Complete ten repetitions
- Perform two sets
- Repeat three to four times per week

Wall Angels

EC14

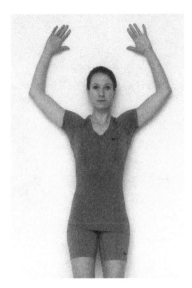

- Stand against a wall with your feet two feet away from the wall and your entire back—from tailbone to head, including the middle of your back—flat against the wall

- Draw your abdominal muscles in, pulling your belly button toward your spine

- Lift your arms over your head with your elbows bent; keep your arms and back flat against the wall

- Begin to move your arms up and down in an arcing motion (as if you're making a snow angel), moving only in the range in which you can keep your back flat against the wall

- Complete ten repetition

- Perform two sets

- Repeat three to four times per week

EC15 | Wall Push-Ups with a Swiss Ball

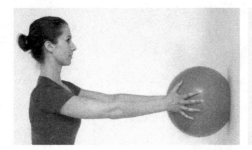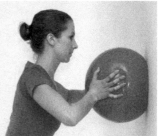

- Place a Swiss ball against a wall slightly below the level of your shoulders
- Extend your arms to hold the ball against the wall and gently squeeze your shoulder blades together and down toward your hips in a "V" position
- Keep your abdominal muscles engaged and your back flat while you bend your elbows, allowing your upper body to move toward the ball as far as comfortably possible until you are in a push-up position
- Push away from the ball, returning to starting position
- Complete ten repetitions
- Perform two sets
- Repeat three to four times per week

Shoulder PNF Stretch

EC16

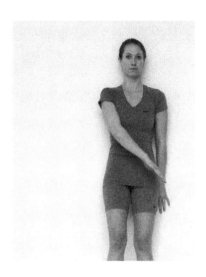
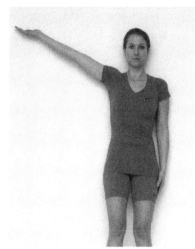

- Stand against a wall with your feet two feet away from the wall and your entire back—from tailbone to head—flat against the wall, including the middle of your back

- Draw your abdominal muscles in, pulling your belly button toward your spine

- Place one arm across your body with your thumb turned toward the opposite pants pocket (your elbow will be slightly bent)

- Gently squeeze your shoulder blade (of the arm you are moving) toward your spine and down toward your hips

- Move with a slow controlled motion, keeping your back flat against the wall throughout the exercise

- Bring your arm up and across your body like you're pulling out a sword; reach your arm up and out and turn your thumb toward the wall, ending with your arm nearly straight and reaching up and away from your body as pictured above

- Complete ten repetitions

- Perform two sets on each arm

- Repeat three to four times per week

Shoulder Circles

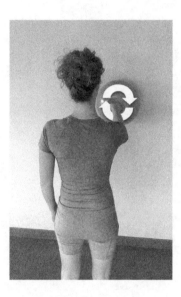

- Stand facing a wall with a ball in front of one shoulder
- Bring your arm up to shoulder level and press your fist into the ball while gently leaning into the ball
- Pull your shoulder blades together and down toward your hips in a "V" position, then use your shoulders to make small circles on the ball
- Complete ten repetitions clockwise, then ten repetitions counter-clockwise
- Perform two sets on each arm
- Repeat three to four times per week

Neck Flexion on Swiss Ball   EC18

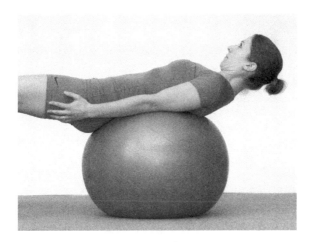

- Lie on a Swiss ball with your back on the ball and your feet on the floor with your knees bent
- Your head should be completely unsupported by the ball (if this position is too difficult or painful, move your body forward on the ball so that your head is supported by the ball)
- Gently tuck your chin into your chest, then raise your head up as though you're trying to touch your chin to the middle of your chest
- Hold for three seconds
- Relax back to neutral position
- Complete ten repetitions
- Repeat in sets of ten repetitions with the goal of reaching thirty repetitions
- Repeat three to four times per week

EC19   Side Flexion on Swiss Ball

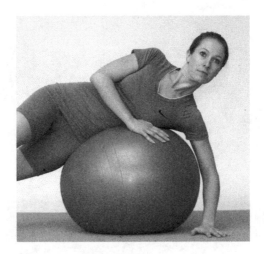

- Lie over a Swiss ball on one side
- Spread your feet apart to provide stability and reach your bottom arm down to touch the floor so that you feel supported
- Keep your ear in line with your shoulder (don't rotate your head during the exercise)
- Complete a side flexion neck lift by bringing your top ear toward your top shoulder
- Hold for three seconds, then return to the neutral position (without support for your head, there will be no rest position)
- Complete ten repetitions
- Repeat in sets of ten repetition with the goal of reaching thirty repetitions
- Repeat the exercise on the other side
- Repeat three to four times per week

Neck Extension on Swiss Ball   EC20

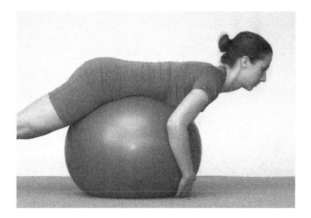

- Position yourself over a Swiss ball so that your stomach is on the ball and your feet are on the floor; if needed, place your hands on the floor for stability (if this position is painful, back your body further onto the ball so that your chin rests on the ball)
- Lift your head, bringing the back of your head toward your feet
- Hold for three seconds
- Relax and return to the starting position
- Complete ten repetitions
- Repeat in sets of ten repetition with the goal of reaching thirty repetitions
- Repeat three to four times per week

Rhomboid "T" on Swiss Ball

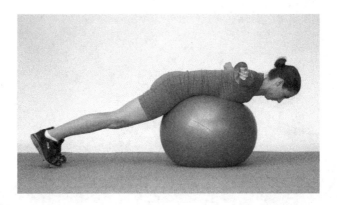

- Lie on a Swiss ball so that your chest and stomach are on the ball and your feet are on the floor with your knees straight
- Be sure to keep your chin slightly tucked and your ears in line with your shoulders to protect your neck
- With thumbs pointing down toward the floor, bring both arms up toward the ceiling until they are parallel with the floor while keeping your elbows straight
- Without raising your arms any higher, gently squeeze your shoulder blades together and down toward your hips
- Hold for three seconds, then relax back into the starting position
- Complete ten repetitions
- Repeat in sets of ten repetitions with the goal of reaching thirty repetitions
- Repeat three to four times per week
- Once you reach your repetitions goal, your provider will show you how to perform this exercise with weights

Middle Trapezius "T" on Swiss Ball EC22

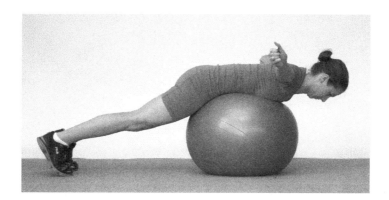

- Lie on a Swiss ball so that your chest and stomach are on the ball and your feet are on the floor with your knees straight

- Be sure to keep your chin slightly tucked and your ears in line with your shoulders to protect your neck

- With thumbs pointing up toward the ceiling, bring both arms up toward the ceiling until they are parallel with the floor while keeping your elbows straight

- Without raising your arms any higher, gently squeeze your shoulder blades together and down toward your hips

- Hold for three seconds, then relax back into the starting position

- Complete ten repetitions

- Repeat in sets of ten repetitions with the goal of reaching thirty repetitions

- Repeat three to four times per week

- Once you reach your repetitions goal, your provider will show you how to perform this exercise with weights

EC23 Lower Trapezius "Y" on Swiss Ball

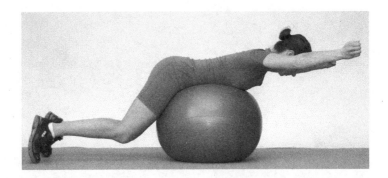

- Lie on a Swiss ball so that your stomach is on the ball with your chest slightly elevated and your feet on the floor with your knees slightly bent
- Be sure to keep your chin slightly tucked and your ears in line with your shoulders to protect your neck
- Move your arms forward until they are in a "Y" position with your thumbs pointing up toward the ceiling
- Gently squeeze your shoulder blades together and down toward your hips in a "V" motion, then raise your arms up toward the ceiling
- Hold for three seconds, then relax back into the starting position
- Complete ten repetitions
- Repeat in sets of ten repetitions with the goal of reaching thirty repetitions
- Repeat three to four times per week
- Once you reach your repetitions goal, your provider will show you how to perform this exercise with weights

Prone Walk-Out

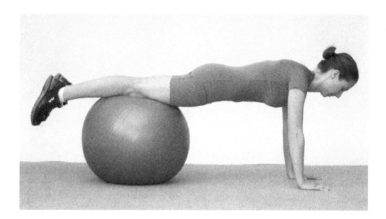

- Begin by kneeling behind a Swiss ball
- Slowly bring yourself up and over the ball by placing your hands on the ground and walking yourself over the ball with your hands
- Your legs should remain on top of the ball
- Continue walking out as far as is comfortably challenging
- Gently squeeze your shoulder blades together and down toward your hips, and keep your abdominal muscles engaged so that your body is flat from your heels to your head (keeping your hips up)
- Keep the exercise pain free
- Hold for ten seconds, then slowly walk yourself back until you are at the starting position
- Complete ten repetitions
- Perform one set
- Repeat three to four times per week

EC25 Prone Push-Ups on Swiss Ball

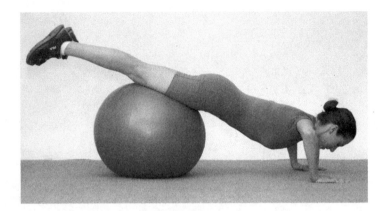

- Begin by kneeling behind a Swiss ball
- Slowly bring yourself up and over the ball by placing your hands on the ground and walking yourself over the ball with your hands
- Your legs should remain on top of the ball
- Continue walking out as far as is comfortably challenging
- Keep your abdominal muscles tight and engaged so that your body is flat from your head to your feet
- Gently squeeze your shoulder blades together and down toward your hips, then bend your elbows and lower yourself into a push-up position only as deep as you are comfortable
- Push your body back up into starting position
- Complete ten repetitions, then return to your knees resting behind the ball
- Perform two sets
- Repeat three to four times per week

Side Plank

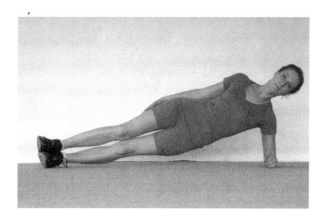

- Begin by lying on your side
- Place your elbow directly under your shoulder with your elbow, forearm, and hand resting comfortably on the floor for support
- Keep your abdominal muscles engaged and your body straight from your head to your heels
- Lift your hips up off the floor three inches, trying to get in line from your shoulders to your feet
- Hold for ten seconds
- Return to the starting position and rest
- Complete five repetitions
- Perform two sets
- Repeat three to four times per week

Plank Twists

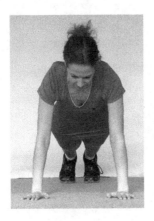 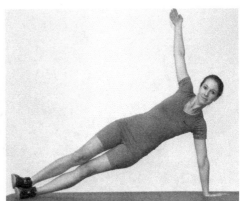

- Starting in a standard plank position on the floor with your hands directly below your shoulders, your head in line with your body, your knees locked straight, and your hips in line with your spine, make sure you're pulling your belly button toward your spine

- Hold for ten seconds

- Start to shift your weight toward one hand; while keeping your abdominal muscles engaged, twist your spine in a slow, controlled way until you are reaching up toward the ceiling as pictured above (keeping your body in a straight line)

- Hold for ten seconds

- Rotate back down to the starting position and hold for ten seconds

- Shift toward the other hand and twist to the other direction, holding for ten seconds

- End in the starting position and rest

- Complete five repetitions

- Perform two sets

- Repeat three to four times per week

Pelvic Tilts

EL1

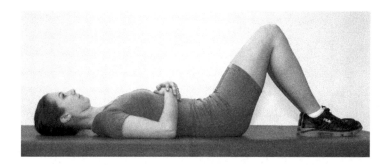

- Lie on your back with your knees bent and your feet flat on the floor
- Draw your abdominal muscles in, pulling your belly button toward your spine while continuing to breathe
- Hold for ten seconds
- Rest and allow your muscles to relax
- Complete ten repetitions
- Perform two sets
- Perform once per day

EL2

Pelvic Tilts with One Leg Up

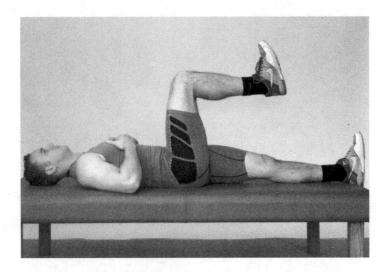

- Lie on your back with your legs straight
- Draw your abdominal muscles in, pulling your belly button toward your spine while continuing to breathe
- While maintaining the contraction of your abdominal muscles, bring one knee up to 90 degrees and then slowly lower it back to the starting position
- Repeat on the other side, then relax
- Complete ten repetitions on each side
- Perform two sets per leg
- Repeat three to four times per week

Isometric Abdominal Contraction EL3

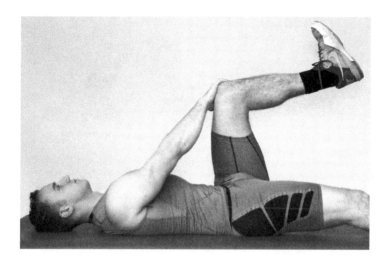

- Lie on your back with your legs straight
- Draw your abdominal muscles in, pulling your belly button toward your spine while continuing to breathe
- While maintaining the contraction of your abdominal muscles, bring one knee up to 90 degrees (as pictured above)
- With your knee at 90 degrees, apply pressure with the opposite hand and match the resistance with your knee by tightening your abdominal muscles
- Hold for five seconds
- Keeping your abdominal muscles tight, slowly lower your leg to starting position
- Repeat on the other leg
- Complete ten repetitions on each side
- Perform two sets per leg
- Repeat three to four times per week

EL4

Bridge

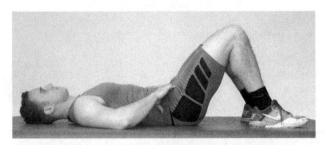

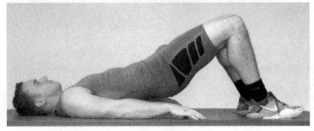

- Lie on your back with your knees bent and your feet flat on the floor
- Place your arms at your sides for stability
- Perform a pelvic tilt by pulling your belly button toward your spine to engage your abdominal muscles
- Tighten your gluteal muscles and raise your hips off the floor
- Your shoulders should remain in contact with the floor
- Do not engage your lower back muscles
- Hold for ten seconds, then slowly lower your hips back to the starting position, relaxing your abdominal muscles last
- Complete ten repetitions
- Perform two sets
- Repeat three to four times per week

Cross-Crawl

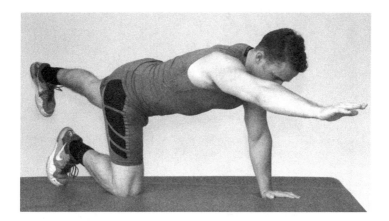

- Kneel on your hands and knees with your hands under your shoulders and your knees under your hips
- Engage your abdominal muscles by pulling your belly button toward your spine
- While holding this position, slowly extend your left leg behind you and your right arm in front of you while keeping your back straight (do not raise either your leg or your arm higher than parallel with the floor)
- Hold for five seconds, then lower your arm and leg to the starting position and relax
- Repeat the exercise on the opposite side
- Complete ten repetitions on each side
- Perform two sets
- Repeat three to four times per week

EL6 Bridge with Leg Extension

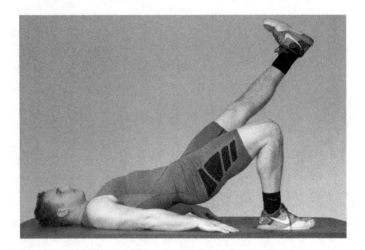

- Lie on your back with your knees bent and your feet flat on the floor
- Place your arms at your sides for stability
- Engage your abdominal muscles by pulling your belly button toward your spine
- Tighten your gluteal muscles and raise your hips off the floor
- Once your hips are elevated, extend one leg straight while keeping your hips level
- Hold for five seconds
- Place your foot back on the floor and extend the other leg while keeping your hips up in the air
- Hold for five seconds on the other leg
- Place your foot back on the floor and lower your hips back to the starting position
- Relax your abdominal muscles
- Complete ten repetitions
- Perform two sets
- Repeat three to four times per week

Theraband Hip Extension   EL7

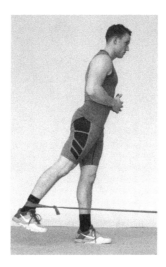

- Place a Theraband in a door (hinge side) about four inches above the floor
- Place the Theraband loop around your ankle and face the door
- Stand straight and tighten your abdominal muscles by pulling your belly button toward your spine
- Keeping the leg with the Theraband straight, extend it backward about twelve inches without leaning forward
- Hold for five seconds
- Slowly move back to the starting position and relax
- Complete ten repetitions on each side
- Perform two sets
- Repeat three to four times per week
- You can use a broom or stick for support if needed, but make sure you stand tall without leaning forward

EL8

Theraband Hip Abduction

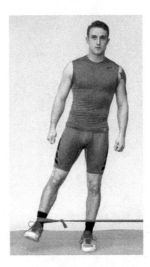

- Place a Theraband in a door (hinge side) about four inches above the floor
- Stand perpendicular to the door
- Place the Theraband loop around the ankle that's furthest from the door
- Stand straight and tighten your abdominal muscles by pulling your belly button toward your spine
- Keeping the leg with the Theraband straight, bring it away from your body and out toward the side about twelve inches
- Avoid pointing your toes outward during the exercise
- Hold for five seconds
- Slowly move back to the starting position and relax
- Complete ten repetitions on each side
- Perform two sets
- Repeat three to four times per week
- You can use a broom or stick for support if needed, but make sure you stand tall without leaning forward

Theraband Hip Flexion   EL9

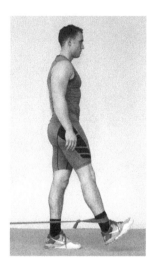

- Place a Theraband in a door (hinge side) about four inches above the floor
- Place the Theraband loop around your ankle and face away from the door
- Stand straight and tighten your abdominal muscles by pulling your belly button toward your spine
- Keeping the leg with the Theraband straight, kick it forward about twelve inches without leaning forward
- Hold for five seconds
- Slowly move back to the starting position and relax
- Complete ten repetitions on each side
- Perform two sets
- Repeat three to four times per week
- You can use a broom or stick for support if needed, but make sure you stand tall without leaning forward

EL10 # Theraband Hip Adduction

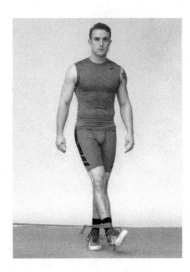

- Place a Theraband in a door (hinge side) about four inches above the floor
- Stand perpendicular to the door
- Place the Theraband loop around the ankle that's nearest to the door
- Stand straight and tighten your abdominal muscles by pulling your belly button toward your spine
- Keeping the leg with the Theraband straight, cross the midline of your body about twelve inches without twisting your spine
- Hold for five seconds
- Slowly move back to the starting position and relax
- Complete ten repetitions
- Perform two sets
- Repeat three to four times per week
- You can use a broom or stick for support if needed, but make sure you stand tall without leaning forward

Up Crunches

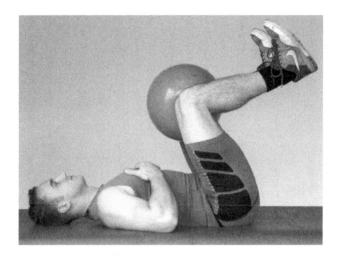

- Lie on your back on the floor
- Place a Swiss ball or folded pillow between your knees and gently squeeze
- Engage your abdominal muscles by pulling your belly button toward your spine
- Bring your knees up to 90 degrees at your hips
- While maintaining the contraction of your abdominal muscle, bring your knees toward your chest three inches, engaging your upper abdominal muscles to "crunch" your knees toward your chest without raising your head or shoulders
- Return your knees to the level of your hips
- Complete ten repetitions, then relax and place your feet on the floor to rest
- Perform two sets
- Repeat three to four times per week

Down Crunches

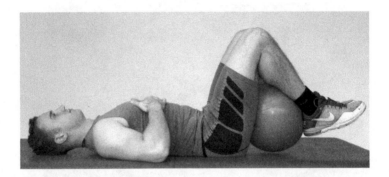

- Lie on your back on the floor
- Place a Swiss ball or folded pillow under your knees and gently squeeze
- Engage your abdominal muscles by pulling your belly button toward your spine
- Bring your knees up to 90 degrees at your hips
- Slowly lower your legs toward the floor, moving two inches while keeping your back flat on the mat
- Pull your knees back up to the level of your hips
- Complete ten repetitions, then relax and place your feet on the floor to rest
- Perform two sets
- Repeat three to four times per week

Abdominal Bicycle

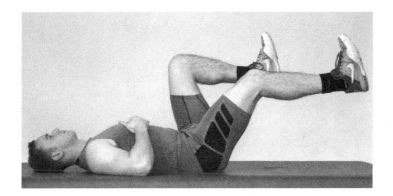

- Lie on your back on the floor
- Engage your abdominal muscles by pulling your belly button toward your spine
- Bring both your knees up to 90 degrees at your hips
- While maintaining the contraction of your abdominal muscles, slowly extend one leg away from your body while holding the other leg in the starting position
- As you draw your first leg back to the starting position, extend the opposite leg
- Alternate legs in a back and forth motion while maintaining a regular breathing pattern and a flat back
- Complete ten repetitions on each side, then rest by bringing your feet back to the floor
- Perform two sets
- Repeat three to four times per week

EL14 Seated Pelvic Tilts on Swiss Ball

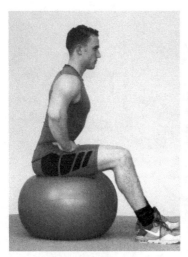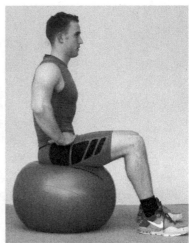

- Sit on a Swiss ball with your weight over the center of the ball and your arms relaxed

- Engage your abdominal muscles by drawing your belly button in toward your spine and rotate your pelvis backward as if you are tucking your "tail" beneath you (your upper body should remain fairly still)

- Hold this position for five seconds

- Allow your abdominal muscles to relax and your pelvis to rotate forward for five seconds

- The ball may shift forward and backward slightly with activation and relaxation of your abdominal muscles, but avoid using your legs

- Complete ten repetitions in each position

- Perform two sets

- Perform once per day

Side Tilts on Swiss Ball

EL15

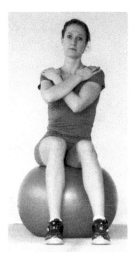 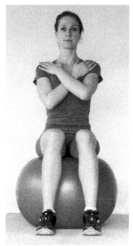 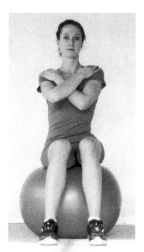

- Sit on a Swiss ball with your weight over the center of the ball and your arms relaxed

- Engage your abdominal muscles by pulling your belly button toward your spine

- Raise one hip up as if to bring your hip and rib cage (on the same side of your body) closer together

- Hold for five seconds

- Tilt to the opposite side, holding that position for five seconds

- Your upper body should remain fairly still

- The ball may roll slightly from side to side, but avoid using your legs

- Complete ten repetitions in each position

- Perform two sets

- Perform once per day

Sit and Bounce

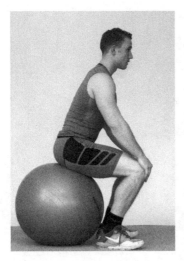 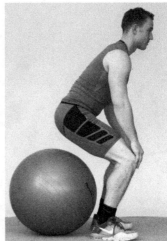

- Sit on a Swiss ball with your weight over the center of the ball and your arms relaxed

- Engage your abdominal muscles by pulling your belly button toward your spine

- Gently bounce up (about six inches) and down on the ball while maintaining the contraction of your abdominal muscles and a neutral spine, keeping your movement controlled and centered over the ball

- Bounce for two minutes

- Perform once per day

Seated March

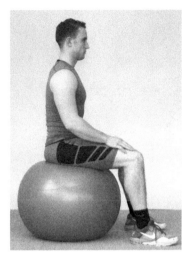 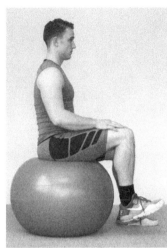

- Sit on a Swiss ball with your weight over the center of the ball and your arms relaxed

- Place your feet shoulder-width apart

- Engage your abdominal muscles by pulling your belly button toward your spine

- Raise one foot three inches off the floor, hold for five seconds, then return it to the floor

- Raise the opposite foot off the floor, hold for five seconds, then return it to the floor

- Complete ten repetitions on each leg

- Perform two sets

- Perform once per day

- To increase the difficulty of the exercise, lift the opposite arm toward the ceiling at the same time the foot comes off the floor

EL18 # Supine Bridge on Swiss Ball

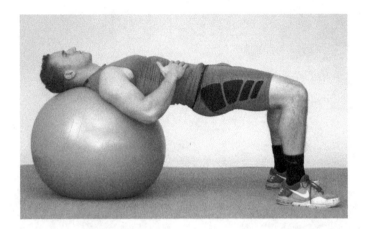

- Sit on a Swiss ball with your weight over the center of the ball and your arms relaxed

- Engage your abdominal muscles by pulling your belly button toward your spine

- Slowly walk your feet forward and let your body roll down with the ball until your head and shoulders are resting on the ball

- Your knees should be bent to 90 degrees with your feet flat on the floor

- Squeeze your gluteal muscles to bring your hips in line with your knees and shoulders

- Hold this position for ten seconds

- Keeping your abdominal muscles engaged, slowly start to walk back toward the ball; when your low back is over the ball, begin to "crunch"; roll your body back into the starting position and rest

- Complete ten repetitions

- Perform two sets

- Repeat three to four times per week

Supine Hip Lifts

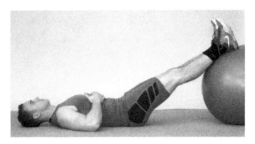

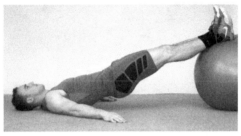

- Lie on your back with your heels supported on a Swiss ball
- Keep your knees straight and your arms at your sides for stability
- Engage your abdominal muscles by pulling your belly button toward your spine
- Squeeze your gluteal muscles and push your heels into the ball to lift your hips off the floor until you are in line with your trunk
- Hold this position for ten seconds, then lower yourself back to the floor and rest
- Complete ten repetitions
- Perform two sets
- Repeat three to four times per week
- To increase the difficulty, place your hands on your stomach or cross your arms over your chest
- Once you have mastered this exercise with both your heels on the ball, challenge yourself to complete it with one ankle crossed over the other, holding that position for ten seconds; complete five repetitions with each leg

Cross-Crawl on a Swiss Ball

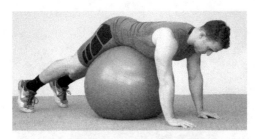

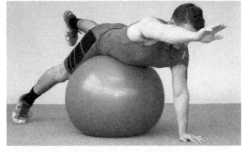

- Position yourself over a Swiss ball so that your stomach is on the ball and your feet and hands are touching the floor

- Engage your abdominal muscles by pulling your belly button toward your spine

- Slowly extend one leg behind you, lifting it off the floor; extend the opposite hand out in front of you until both your leg and your hand are parallel with the level of your trunk

- Hold for ten seconds, then lower your arm and leg back to the starting position

- Repeat with the opposite arm and leg, re-engaging your abdominal muscles before you move.

- Complete ten repetitions on each side

- Perform two sets

- Repeat three to four times per week

Bridge with Leg Extension   EL21

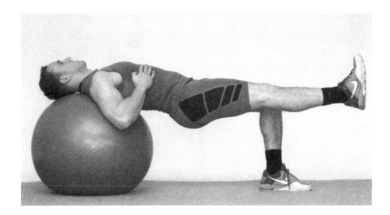

- Sit on a Swiss ball with your weight over the center of the ball and your arms relaxed

- Engage your abdominal muscles by pulling your belly button toward your spine

- Slowly walk your feet forward and let your body roll down with the ball until your head and shoulders are resting on the ball

- Continue to engage your abdominal muscles while squeezing your gluteal muscles to keep your hips at the level of your trunk

- Raise one leg up parallel to the ground at the height of your body level

- Hold for five seconds, then return your foot to the floor and perform the same movement with the opposite leg

- Complete ten repetitions on each side, then slowly start to walk back toward the ball, finally rolling back up to the starting position

- Perform two sets

- Repeat three to four times per week

EL22 Hip Lift with Straight Leg Raises

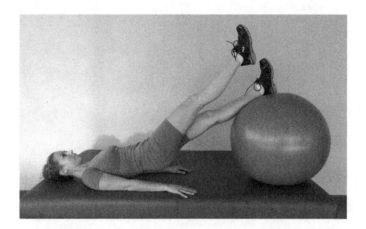

- Lie on your back with your heels supported on a Swiss ball
- Keep your knees straight and your arms at your sides for stability
- Engage your abdominal muscles by pulling your belly button toward your spine
- Squeeze your gluteal muscles and push your heels into the ball to lift your hips off the floor
- While maintaining this position, lift one of your legs twelve inches off the ball
- Hold for five seconds, return that heel to the ball, then perform the same movement with the opposite leg
- Bring your leg back down to the ball, then lower your hips to the floor and rest
- Complete ten repetitions
- Perform two sets
- Repeat three to four times per week
- To increase the difficulty, place your arms across your chest

Crunches on Swiss Ball   EL23

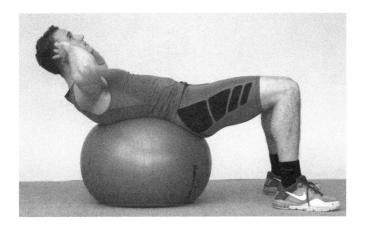

- Start by sitting on a Swiss ball
- Take a step forward and roll yourself down until the small of your back is resting on the ball and your shoulders and head are unsupported
- Keep your back in a neutral position with your hands behind your neck; tuck your chin to protect your neck
- Perform a one-to-two inch curl up from the ball, leading with your chest toward the ceiling
- Hold for three seconds
- Lower yourself back to the starting position
- Complete ten repetitions, then return to the starting position and rest
- Perform two sets
- Repeat three to four times per week
- You can perform oblique crunches in the same manner by slightly rotating your spine to the left or right at the top of the curl-up

Knee Tucks

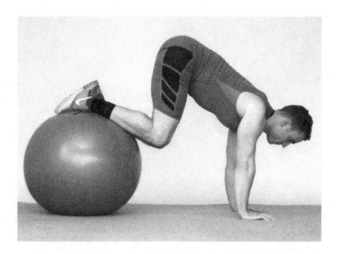

- Begin by kneeling behind a Swiss ball
- Slowly bring yourself up and over the ball by placing your hands on the ground and walking yourself over the ball until your shins are resting on the ball
- Engage your abdominal muscles by pulling your belly button toward your spine
- Draw your knees in toward your chest, allowing the ball to roll with your legs
- Hold for three seconds, then return to the flat position while continuing to engage your abdominal muscles
- Perform ten repetitions, then roll yourself back to the starting position and rest
- Perform two sets
- Repeat three to four times per week

Skiers

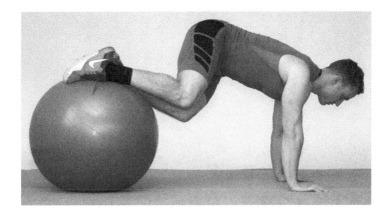

- Begin by kneeling behind a Swiss ball
- Slowly bring yourself up and over the ball by placing your hands on the ground and walking yourself over the ball until your shins are resting on the ball
- Engage your abdominal muscles by pulling your belly button toward your spine
- While keeping your abdominal muscles engaged, rotate your hips toward the right, then pull your knees toward your right shoulder, enabling your pelvis to rotate
- Return to neutral position, then perform the same movement on the left side
- Repeat five times on each side, then walk back to the starting position and rest
- Perform two sets
- Repeat three to four times per week

Double Leg Lift

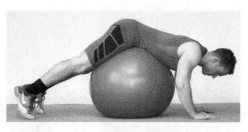

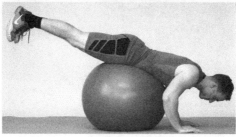

- Lie on your stomach over the ball with the ball positioned below your hips
- Place your hands on the floor with your elbows slightly bent and your head down (similar to a push-up position)
- Keep your legs straight and feet together
- Engage your abdominal muscles by pulling your belly button toward your spine
- While squeezing your gluteal muscles, lift your legs until they are in line with your body
- Hold for ten seconds, then lower your legs down to the floor and rest
- Complete ten repetitions
- Perform two sets
- Repeat three to four times per week

Pikes on Swiss Ball

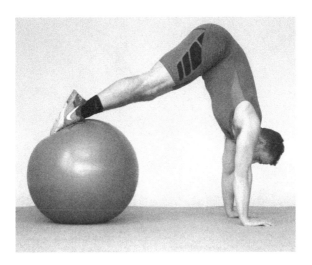

- Start by kneeling behind a Swiss ball on the floor
- Slowly bring yourself up and over the ball by placing your hands on the ground and walking yourself over the ball until your ankles are resting on the ball
- Keeping your abdominal muscles engaged and your knees straight and ankles relaxed, lift your hips into the air as pictured above
- The ball should move toward your hands as you raise your hips
- Hold this position for three seconds, then return to a flat position
- Repeat ten times, then roll back to the starting position while continuing to engage your abdominal muscles
- Complete ten repetitions, then roll yourself back to the starting position and rest
- Perform two sets
- Repeat three to four times per week

EL28 | Single Leg Hamstring Curls

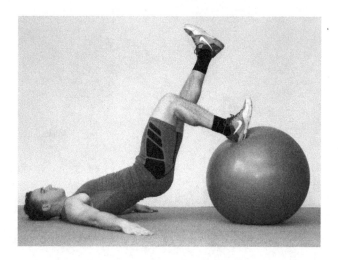

- Lie on your back with your heels supported on a Swiss ball
- Keep your knees straight and your arms at your sides for stability
- Engage your abdominal muscles by pulling your belly button in toward your spine
- Squeeze your gluteal muscles and push your heels into the ball to lift your hips off the floor
- Lift one leg off the ball and maintain it in the air throughout the entire exercise
- Bend the knee of the supporting leg that is on the ball and pull the ball toward your hips with your heel
- Slowly return to the starting position
- Complete ten repetitions, then place your other leg back onto the ball and lower your hips to the floor
- Repeat the exercise with your other leg
- Perform two sets per leg
- Repeat three to four times per week

Dead Bug

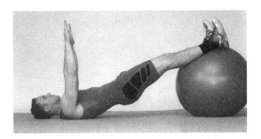

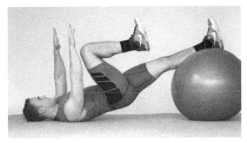

- Lie on your back with your heels supported on a Swiss ball
- Keep your knees straight and your arms up in the air as pictured above
- Engage your abdominal muscles by pulling your belly button in toward your spine
- Squeeze your gluteal muscles and push your heels into the ball to lift your hips off the floor
- Keeping your hips up in the air, lift one leg off the ball and slowly bend your knee back toward your elbow on the same side
- Place that leg back onto the ball
- Keeping your hips in the air, lift the opposite leg and bring it toward the same-side elbow
- Complete ten repetitions on each leg, then lower your hips to the floor and relax
- Perform two sets
- Repeat three to four times per week

EL30

Single Knee Tucks

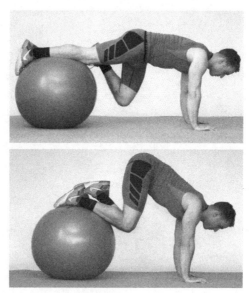

- Begin by kneeling behind a Swiss ball

- Slowly bring yourself up and over the ball by placing your hands on the ground and walking yourself over the ball until it is resting under your shins

- Engage your abdominal muscles by pulling your belly button in toward your spine

- Draw one of your knees toward your chest and hold it clear of the ball while the other leg remains straight and supported on the ball as pictured above

- With the supporting leg still on the ball, pull that knee toward your chest, rolling the ball toward your head, then return to the starting position

- Perform ten repetitions with the same leg, then roll back to the starting position

- Repeat the exercise with the opposite leg

- Perform two sets

- Repeat three to four times per week

Froggies

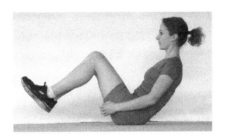

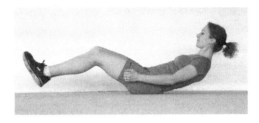

- Start by sitting on the floor
- Engage your abdominal muscles by pulling your belly button in toward your spine
- Roll back onto your buttocks so that you are able to maintain your balance with your feet off the floor
- Keeping your abdominal muscles engaged, slowly lower your trunk toward the floor while extending your feet out away from your body
- If you are able to, reach your arms over your head while you are leaning back
- Return to the starting position
- Complete ten repetitions
- Perform two sets
- Repeat three to four times per week
- The goal is to be able to complete ten repetitions without touching your feet to the floor; however, if needed, you can touch your feet to the floor to rest

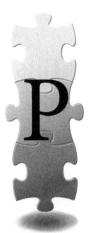

Proprioceptive Training Exercises

The most advanced form of stabilization exercises included in your DMR Method program are called Proprioceptive Training Exercises. Sensors throughout your joints and ligaments, called proprioceptors, respond to movement and send that information to the brain. Your brain uses this information to help maintain normal posture, alignment, and balance in your body. Long-term mobility and alignment issues cause a disruption in healthy proprioception. This leads to instability, poor coordination, and imbalance. Proprioceptive Training Exercises help you rebuild this part of your nervous system and are a key to optimal recovery. On the next few pages you will learn many of the DMR Method Proprioceptive Training Exercises that may be used to help enhance proprioception and stability.

P1   Seated Pelvic Tilts on Swiss Ball

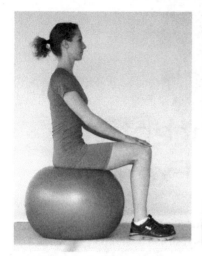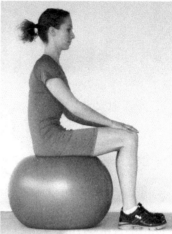

- Sit on a Swiss ball with your weight over the center of the ball and your arms relaxed

- Engage your abdominal muscles by drawing your belly button toward your spine as if you are tucking your tailbone beneath you (your upper body should remain fairly still)

- Hold this position for five seconds

- Allow your abdominal muscles to relax and your pelvis to rotate forward for five seconds

- The ball may shift forward and backward slightly with activation and relaxation of your abdominal muscles, but avoid using your legs

- Complete ten repetitions in each position

- Perform two sets

- Perform once per day

Seated Side Tilts on Swiss Ball   P2

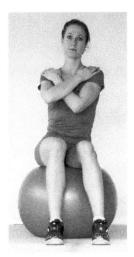 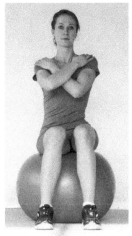 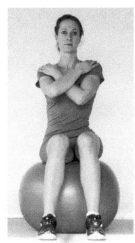

- Sit on a Swiss ball with your weight over the center of the ball and your arms crossed

- Focus on keeping your upper body still during this exercise, only using your legs to maintain balance

- Engage your abdominal muscles by pulling your belly button toward your spine

- Raise one hip up as if to bring your hip and rib cage (on the same side of your body) closer together

- Hold for five seconds

- Repeat the same procedure on the opposite side

- Repeat ten times in each direction

- Perform two sets

- Perform once per day

P3

Seated Bounce on Swiss Ball

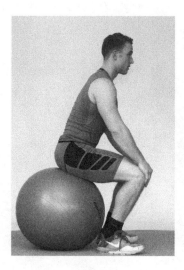 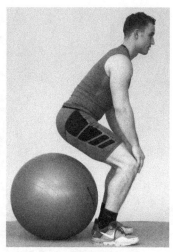

- Sit on a Swiss ball with your weight over the center of the ball and your arms relaxed

- Place your feet shoulder-width apart

- Engage your abdominal muscles by pulling your belly button toward your spine

- Gently bounce up (about twelve inches) and down on the ball while maintaining the contraction of your abdominal muscles and a neutral spine, keeping your movement controlled and centered over the ball

- Bounce for two minutes

- Perform once per day

Seated March on Swiss Ball

P4

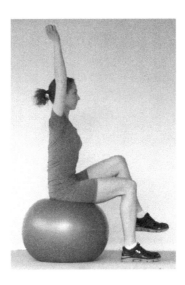

- Sit on a Swiss ball with your weight over the center of the ball and your arms relaxed

- Place your feet shoulder-width apart

- Engage your abdominal muscles by pulling your belly button toward your spine

- Raise one foot three inches off the floor while simultaneously raising your opposite arm up toward the ceiling; hold for five seconds, then return your foot to the floor and relax your arm

- Repeat with the opposite knee and arm, keeping your abdominal muscles engaged throughout the exercise

- Complete ten repetitions on each side

- Perform two sets

- Perform once per day

Tandem Stance

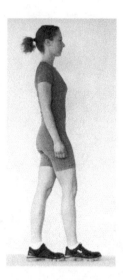

- Place your right foot directly in front of your left foot so that you are toe to heel as pictured above

- Stand in good upright posture with your abdominal muscles engaged and your knees slightly bent

- Hold for one minute, then repeat the exercise with your left foot in front of your right for one minute

- If needed, hold onto a counter or railing, but use only as much pressure with your hands as needed for safety; the goal is to complete this exercise without external support

- Perform once per day

- If approved by your provider, you can make this exercise more challenging by performing it with your eyes closed

Narrow Base of Support   **P6**

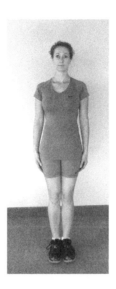

- Stand with your feet as close together as possible in good upright posture with a slight bend in your knees
- Engage your abdominal muscles by pulling your belly button toward your spine
- Hold for one minute
- If needed, hold onto a counter or railing, but use only as much pressure with your hands as needed for safety; the goal is to complete this exercise without external support
- Perform once per day
- If approved by your provider, you can make this exercise more challenging by performing it with your eyes closed

Single Leg Stance

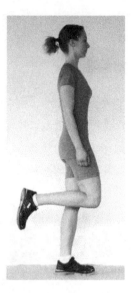

- Put all of your weight on one foot and bend your other knee until your lower leg is parallel to the floor

- Maintain a small bend in your weight-bearing leg and stand tall with your abdominal muscles engaged

- Hold in this position with your eyes open for one minute

- If needed, hold onto a counter or railing, but use only as much pressure with your hands as needed for safety; the goal is to complete this exercise without external support

- Return your foot to the floor, rest, then repeat the exercise with the other leg

- Perform once per day

- If approved by your provider, you can make this exercise more challenging by performing it with your eyes closed

Single Leg Stance with Flexion   P8

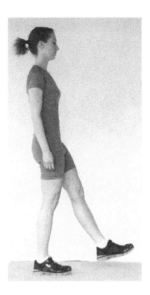

- Put all of your weight on one foot

- Maintain a small bend in your weight-bearing leg and stand tall with your abdominal muscles engaged

- Keeping your non-supported leg straight, bring it out in front of you twelve inches off the floor

- Hold this position with your eyes open for thirty seconds, then return your foot back to the floor and relax

- Complete five repetitions

- If needed, hold onto a counter or railing, but use only as much pressure with your hands as needed for safety; the goal is to complete this exercise without external support

- Repeat the exercise with the opposite leg

- Perform once per day

- If approved by your provider, you can make this exercise more challenging by performing it with your eyes closed

P9 Single Leg Stance with Abduction

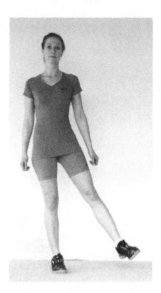

- Put all of your weight on one foot
- Maintain a small bend in your weight-bearing leg and stand tall with your abdominal muscles engaged
- Keeping your non-supported leg straight, bring it out to the side twelve inches
- Hold this position with your eyes open for thirty seconds, then return your foot back to the floor and relax
- Complete five repetitions
- If needed, hold onto a counter or railing, but use only as much pressure with your hands as needed for safety; the goal is to complete this exercise without external support
- Repeat the exercise with the opposite leg
- Perform once per day
- If approved by your provider, you can make this exercise more challenging by performing it with your eyes closed

Double Leg Balance

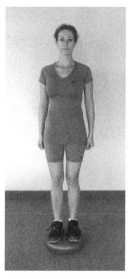 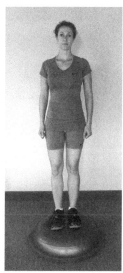

- Place a Dynadisc or BOSU ball on the floor, flat side down, in front of a counter, railing, or supportive piece of furniture
- Hold onto the support structure while stepping onto the equipment to avoid losing your balance
- Stand with your feet hip-width apart with a slight bend in your knees
- Engage your abdominal muscles by pulling your belly button toward your spine
- Hold for one minute
- If needed hold onto the support structure during the exercise, but use only as much pressure with your hands as needed for safety; the goal is to complete this exercise without external support
- Perform once per day

Single Leg Balance

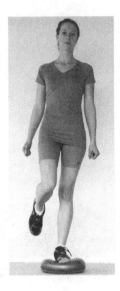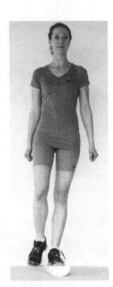

- Place a half-foam roll, Dynadisc, or BOSU ball on the floor, flat side down, in front of a counter, railing, or supportive piece of furniture

- Hold onto the support structure while stepping onto the equipment to avoid losing your balance

- Engage your abdominal muscles by pulling your belly button toward your spine

- Stand with all your weight on one leg, slightly bending that knee with your foot in the middle of the piece of equipment

- If needed hold onto the support structure during the exercise, but use only as much pressure with your hands as needed for safety; the goal is to complete this exercise without external support

- Hold for thirty seconds then step down and rest

- Complete three repetitions

- Repeat the exercise with the other foot

- Perform once per day

Lunge

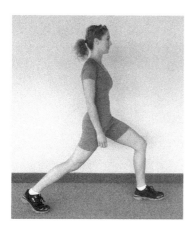 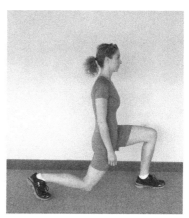

- Standing upright with good posture, engage your abdominal muscles by pulling your belly button toward your spine
- Step forward with your left leg so that your foot is two feet in front of your right foot; ensure that both feet are pointing straight ahead
- Slowly lower yourself straight down toward the floor (making sure to keep your left knee behind your left toes) twelve inches, then slowly return to standing position
- Complete ten repetitions
- Return to the starting position and rest
- Repeat the exercise with your other foot
- Perform two sets per side
- Repeat three to four times per week

P13

Advanced Lunge

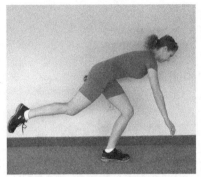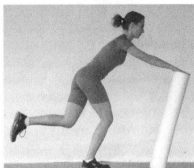

- Standing upright with good posture, engage your abdominal muscles by pulling your belly button toward your spine
- Step forward with your left leg so that your foot is two feet in front of your right foot; ensure that both feet are pointing straight ahead
- Raise your back leg off the floor
- Slowly lower yourself straight down toward the floor (making sure to keep your left knee behind your left toes) twelve inches, then slowly return to standing position
- Complete ten repetitions
- Return to the starting position and rest
- Repeat the exercise with your other foot
- Perform two sets per side
- Repeat three to four times per week
- It may be necessary to use a stick or other support at first, but the goal is to perform this maneuver without external support

Squat on BOSU

P14

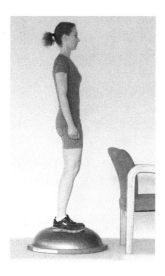
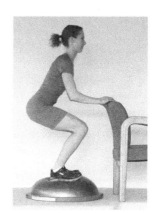

- Position a BOSU ball with the flat side facing down
- Holding onto a counter or railing, climb onto the BOSU ball with your feet shoulder-width apart
- Engage your abdominal muscles by pulling your belly button toward your spine
- Bring your hips back as if you were going to sit in a chair; lower yourself down while bending your knees twelve inches, then return to the starting position and rest
- Hold onto a counter or railing only as much as you need to in order to feel safe while lowering your body
- Complete ten repetitions
- Perform two sets
- Repeat three to four times per week
- For an added challenge, this exercise can be completed with the flat side of the BOSU facing up

P15 Prone Walkout with Hand March

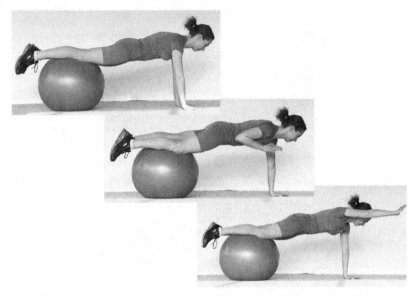

- Begin by kneeling behind a Swiss ball.
- Slowly bring yourself up and over the ball by placing your hands on the ground and walking yourself over the ball until your shins are resting on the ball
- Maintaining this position, slowly raise one hand off the floor six inches, then immediately return it to the floor
- As you get stronger, work up to lifting your hand off the floor twelve to eighteen inches and holding it for five seconds; then progress to reaching your hand out straight in front of you and holding it for five seconds
- Maintain form and try not to shift your weight
- Repeat the exercise with your other hand
- Perform ten repetitions on each side
- Roll back on the ball and return to the starting position to rest
- Perform two sets
- Repeat three to four times per week
- If you are unable to maintain proper form, back up further on the ball to make the exercise easier

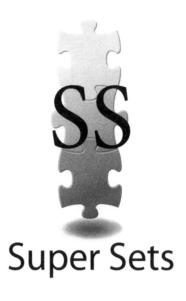

Super Sets

Fast, Fun, Effective Conditioning!

As the DMR Method clinical case study research has shown, a key to short-term and long-term recovery is consistency with the stabilization component of the DMR Method. This is especially true in the first few months after completing the clinical care elements. Remember the eleven-to-eighteen month rule: even with complete resolution of all symptoms, it takes the supportive soft tissues eleven to eighteen months to heal completely! During this time frame, it's essential that you continually and consistently reinforce your correction with the right stabilization procedures. To supplement the body mechanics training, stretching, and exercises that were designed specifically for your condition, DMR Method providers have designed a number of five-minute Super Sets that are a fast, fun, and effective way to optimize the stabilization component of your program. We've even designed workouts that you can do at work and when you're on vacation! All of these workouts include spine-healthy stretching and conditioning exercises that can be performed anywhere in less than ten minutes. Your DMR Method provider will help you select the Super Set workouts that are best for you. Make sure when using these workouts that you continue to follow any restrictions and honor any physical limitations that you may have discussed with your DMR Method provider. If you'd like to do your five-minute Super Set workouts with a trainer, you can follow along with videos at:

DMRMethod.com/Patient Resources/SuperSetWorkouts

Super Set #1: Cervical

SS1

- **Upper Trapezius Stretch** (SC1, page 152). Sit with good posture. Keeping your nose pointing straight ahead, tilt your head to bring one ear straight down toward your shoulder until you feel a good stretch. Hold for forty-five to sixty seconds. Gently return to neutral position, then repeat the stretch on the other side. Complete one repetition on each side.

- **Levator Stretch** (SC2, page 153). Sit with good posture. Turn your head 45 degrees, then bring your nose down toward the same armpit until you feel a stretch on the back side of your neck on the opposite side. Hold for forty-five to sixty seconds. Gently return to neutral position, then repeat the stretch on the other side. Complete one repetition on each side.

- **Chin Tucks/Scapular Sets** (EC1 & EC2, page 186 & 187). Sit or stand with good posture. Bring your arms up to 90 degrees at your shoulders and elbows. Slowly move your chin straight back one to two inches until your ears are in line with your shoulders; simultaneously squeeze your shoulder blades down and together in a "V" position. Hold for five seconds, then rest. Complete five repetitions per set; perform two sets.

- **Wall Angels** (EC14, page 199). Stand against a wall with your feet two feet away from the wall and your entire back—from tailbone to head, including the middle of your back—flat against the wall by drawing your abdominal muscles in. Lift your arms over your head with your elbows bent while keeping your entire arms and back flat against the wall. Begin to move your arms up and down in an arcing motion, moving only in the range in which you can keep your back flat against the wall. Complete ten repetitions per set; perform two sets.

- **Side Plank** (EC26, page 211). Begin by lying on your side. Place your elbow directly under your shoulder with your elbow, forearm, and hand resting comfortably on the floor for support. Keep your abdominal muscles engaged and your body straight from your head to your heels. Lift your hips up off the floor three inches, trying to get in line from your shoulders to your feet. Hold for ten seconds. Return to the starting position and rest. Complete five repetitions per set; perform two sets.

Super Set #2: Thoracic

- **Levator Stretch** (SC2, page 153). Sit with good posture. Turn your head 45 degrees, then bring your nose down toward the same armpit until you feel a stretch on the back side of your neck on the opposite side. Hold for forty-five to sixty seconds. Gently return to neutral position, then repeat the stretch on the other side. Complete one repetition on each side.

- **Rhomboid Gas Pedal** (SC5, page 156). Sit forward on the edge of a chair. Place one foot forward, putting the heel on the ground with your toes slightly up in the air with your other knee bent at 90 degrees. Lean forward, bracing your forearm or chest on your thighs, then grab the outside of the foot on the same side with thumb pointed upwards. Without moving your body, keep holding your foot and push it toward the ground like you are pushing on a gas pedal. Hold for forty-five seconds, then repeat on the other side. Complete one repetition on each side.

- **Prayer Stretch** (SC8, page 159). Start on your hands and knees. Keeping your hands where they are, slowly sit back onto your heels. Gently tuck your head down between your elbows until you feel a stretch at the back of your shoulders or in your back. Hold for forty-five to sixty seconds. Complete one repetition.

- **Side Plank** (EC26, page 211). Begin by lying on your side. Place your elbow directly under your shoulder with your elbow, forearm, and hand resting comfortably on the floor for support. Keep your abdominal muscles engaged and your body straight from your head to your heels. Lift your hips up off the floor three inches, trying to get in line from your shoulders to your feet. Hold for ten seconds. Return to the starting position and rest. Complete five repetitions per set; perform two sets.

- **Wall Push-Ups with Swiss Ball** (EC15, page 200). Place a Swiss ball against a wall slightly below the level of your shoulders. Extend your arms to hold the ball against the wall and gently squeeze your shoulder blades together and down toward your hips in a "V" position. Keep your abdominal muscles engaged and your back flat while you bend your elbows, allowing your upper body to move toward the ball as far as comfortably possible until you are in a push-up position. Push away from the ball, then return to starting position. Complete ten repetitions per set; perform two sets.

Super Set #3: Lumbar

- **Hamstring Supine** (SL7, page 171). Lie on your back on the floor with both knees bent and feet flat on the floor. Place a towel or belt around one foot, keeping it in the arch of the foot. Extend your leg until your knee is straight. Begin to pull the strap toward your head, raising your leg up until you feel a stretch in the back of the leg. Hold for forty-five to sixty seconds. Repeat the stretch with the other leg. Perform one repetition with each leg.

- **Piriformis Stretch on Mat** (SL5, page 169). Lie on your back on the floor with your knees bent and your feet flat on the floor. Cross one leg over the other so that your ankle rests on the opposite knee. Hold the stretch for forty-five to sixty seconds. Complete one repetition.

- **Skiers** (EL25, page 237). Begin by kneeling behind a Swiss ball. Slowly bring yourself up and over the ball by placing your hands on the ground and walking yourself over the ball until your shins are resting on the ball. While keeping your abdominal muscles engaged, rotate your hips toward the right, then pull your knees toward your right shoulder, enabling your pelvis to rotate. Return to neutral position, then perform the same movement on the left side. Repeat five times on each side, then walk back to the starting position to rest. Perform two sets.

- **Dead Bug** (EL29, p. 241). Lie on your back with your heels supported on a Swiss ball. Keep your knees straight and your arms up in the air. Squeeze your gluteal muscles and push your heels into the ball to lift your hips off the floor. Keeping your hips up in the air, lift one leg off the ball and slowly bend your knee back toward your elbow on the same side. Place that leg back onto the ball. Keeping your hips in the air, lift the opposite leg and bring it toward the same-side elbow. Complete five repetitions on each leg, then lower your hips back to the floor and rest. Perform two sets.

- **Crunches on Swiss Ball** (EL23, page 235). Start by sitting on a Swiss ball. Take a step forward and roll yourself down until the small of your back is resting on the ball and your shoulder and head are unsupported. Keep your back in a neutral position with your hands behind your neck. Perform a chin tuck to protect your neck. Perform a one-to-two inch curl up from the ball, lifting your head and shoulders toward the ceiling; hold for three seconds. Lower yourself back to the starting position. Complete ten repetitions, then return to the starting position and rest. Perform two sets.

Super Set #4: Lumbar

- **Hamstring Supine** (SL7, page 171). Lie on your back on the floor with both knees bent and feet flat on the floor. Place a towel or belt around one foot, keeping it in the arch of the foot. Extend your leg until your knee is straight. Begin to pull the strap toward your head, raising your leg up until you feel a stretch in the back of the leg. Hold for forty-five to sixty seconds. Repeat the stretch with the other leg. Perform one repetition with each leg.

- **Piriformis Stretch on Mat** (SL5, page 169). Lie on your back on the floor with your knees bent and your feet flat on the floor. Cross one leg over the other so that your ankle rests on the opposite knee. Hold the stretch for forty-five to sixty seconds. Complete one repetition.

- **Double-Leg Lift** (EL26, page 238) Lie on your stomach over the ball with the ball positioned below your hips. Place your hands on the floor with your elbows slightly bent and your head down (similar to a push-up position). Keep your legs straight and feet together. Engage your abdominal muscles by pulling your belly button toward your spine. While engaging your gluteal muscles, lift your legs until they are in line with your body. Hold for ten seconds, then lower your legs back down to the floor. Complete five repetitions per set; perform one set.

- **Side Plank** (EC26, page 211). Begin by lying on your side. Place your elbow directly under your shoulder with your elbow, forearm, and hand resting comfortably on the floor for support. Keep your abdominal muscles engaged and your body straight from your head to your heels. Lift your hips up off the floor three inches, trying to get in line from your shoulders to your feet. Hold for ten seconds. Return to the starting position and rest. Complete five repetitions per set; perform one set.

- **Pikes on Swiss Ball** (EL27, page 239). Start by kneeling behind a Swiss ball on the floor. Slowly bring yourself up and over the ball by placing your hands on the ground and walking yourself over the ball until your ankles are resting on the ball. Keeping your abdominal muscle engaged, your knees straight, and your ankles relaxed, lift your hips into the air. The ball should move toward your hands as you raise your hips. Hold this position for three seconds, then return to a flat position, continuing to engage your abdominal muscles. Complete five repetitions, then roll yourself back to the starting position. Perform two sets.

Super Set #5: Core

- **Trunk Rotation** (SL4, page 168). Lie on your back on the floor with your knees bent up and your feet together flat on the surface. Keeping your shoulders down, gently drop your knees toward the floor, allowing your feet to rotate off the floor until you feel a gentle stretch Hold for forty-five to sixty seconds. Gently bring your knees back to center to return to the starting position, then rotate to the opposite side and hold for forty-five to sixty seconds. Complete one repetition to each side.

- **Chin Tucks/Scapular Sets** (EC1 & EC2, page 186 & 187). Sit or stand with good posture. Bring your arms up to 90 degrees at your shoulders and elbows. Slowly move your chin straight back one to two inches until your ears are in line with your shoulders; simultaneously squeeze your shoulder blades down and together in a "V" position. Hold for five seconds, then rest. Complete five repetitions per set; perform two sets.

- **Froggies** (EL31, page 243) Start by sitting on the floor. Engage your abdominal muscles by pulling your belly button in toward your spine. Roll back onto your buttocks so that you are able to maintain your balance with your feet off the floor. Keeping your abdominal muscles engaged, slowly lean your trunk back toward the floor while extending your feet out away from your body. Complete ten repetitions per set; perform two sets.

- **Abdominal Bicycle** (EL13, page 225). Lie on your back on the floor. Bring both your knees up to 90 degrees at your hips. Slowly extend one leg away from your body while holding the other leg in the starting position. Alternate legs in a back-and-forth motion while maintaining a regular breathing pattern and a flat back throughout. Complete ten repetitions on each side, then rest by bringing your feet back to the floor. Perform two sets.

- **Prone Push-ups on Swiss Ball** (EC25, page 210). Begin by kneeling behind a Swiss ball. Slowly bring yourself up and over the ball by placing your hands on the ground and walking yourself over the ball with your hands. Gently squeeze your shoulder blades together and down toward your hips, then bend your elbows and lower yourself into a push-up position only as deep as you are comfortable. Push your body back up into starting position. Complete ten repetitions, then return to the starting position and rest. Perform two sets.

Cervical / Thoracic - At Work

- **Upper Trapezius Stretch** (SC1, page 152). Sit with good posture. Keeping your nose pointing straight ahead, tilt your head to bring one ear straight down toward your shoulder until you feel a good stretch. Hold for forty-five to sixty seconds. Gently return to neutral position, then repeat the stretch on the other side. Complete one repetition on each side.

- **Levator Stretch** (SC2, page 153). Sit with good posture. Turn your head 45 degrees, then bring your nose down toward the same armpit until you feel a stretch on the back side of your neck on the opposite side. Keep the stretch pain free. Hold for forty-five to sixty seconds. Gently return to neutral position, then repeat the stretch on the other side. Complete one repetition on each side.

- **Chin Tucks/Scapular Sets** (EC1 & EC2, page 186 & 187). Sit or stand with good posture. Bring your arms up to 90 degrees at your shoulders and elbows. Slowly move your chin straight back one to two inches until your ears are in line with your shoulders; simultaneously squeeze your shoulder blades down and together in a "V" position. Hold for five seconds, then rest. Complete five repetitions per set; perform two sets.

- **Wall Push-Ups** (EC15, page 200- done without the the Swiss ball). Place your hands directly on a wall slightly below the level of your shoulders. Extend your arms and gently squeeze your shoulder blades together and down toward your hips in a "V" position. Keeping your abdominal muscles engaged and your back flat, bend your elbows, allowing your upper body to move toward the wall as far as you comfortably can until you are in a push-up position. Push away from the wall, returning to the starting position. Complete ten repetitions per set; perform two sets.

- **Wall Angels** (EC14, page 199). Stand against a wall with your feet two feet away from the wall and your entire back—from tailbone to head, including the middle of your back—flat against the wall by drawing your abdominal muscles in. Lift your arms over your head with your elbows bent while keeping your entire arms and back flat against the wall. Begin to move your arms up and down in an arcing motion, moving only in the range in which you can keep your back flat against the wall. Complete ten repetitions per set; perform two sets.

Lumbar - At Work

- **Hamstring Seated** (SL8, page 172). Sit on the edge of a chair with good posture. Stretch one leg out in front of you with your heel on the floor and your foot relaxed. The other knee should be bent to 90 degrees with the foot flat on the floor. Keeping your spine straight, lean forward until you feel a gentle stretch in the back of the straight leg. Hold for forty-five to sixty seconds, then repeat the stretch with the other leg. Complete one repetition on each side.

- **Piriformis Seated** (SL6, page 170). Sit with good posture in a chair with both knees bent to 90 degrees and your feet planted on the floor. Cross one ankle over the top of the other knee. Keeping your spine in a neutral position (as if a rod is in your spine), lean forward from the hips until you feel a stretch in the leg that is crossed. Hold for forty-five to sixty seconds, then repeat the stretch with the other leg. Complete one repetition on each side.

- **Single-Leg Stance with Flexion** (P8, page 253).Standing in front of a counter, railing, or piece of furniture, put all your weight on one foot. Maintain a small bend in your weight-bearing leg and stand tall with your abdominal muscles engaged. Keeping your non-supported leg straight, bring it out in front of you twelve inches off the floor. Hold this position with your eyes open for thirty seconds. Return your foot back to the floor and relax. Complete five repetitions. If needed, hold onto a counter or railing, but use only as much pressure with your hands as is needed for safety. The goal is to complete this exercise without external support. Repeat the exercise with the opposite leg. (If approved by your provider, you can make this exercise more challenging by performing it with your eyes closed.)

- **Single-Leg Wall Squats** (Not referenced in the exercise section of book). Stand with your back against the wall and your feet shoulder width apart 2 feet from the wall. Engage your abdominal muscles by pulling your belly button toward your spine until your back is flat against the wall. Start to lower your hips down toward the floor (no more than 90 degrees), ensuring that your knees do not travel in front of your toes. Once you are at 90 degrees, while maintaining the contraction of your abdominal muscles, extend one leg out, hold for ten seconds, then lower that leg back to the floor and extend out the other leg for ten seconds. Place that foot on the floor and return to the starting position. Complete five repetitions.

Cervical / Thoracic - On The Go!

- **Upper Trapezius Stretch** (SC1, page 152). Sit with good posture. Keeping your nose pointing straight ahead, tilt your head to bring one ear straight down toward your shoulder until you feel a good stretch. Keep the stretch pain free. Hold for forty-five to sixty seconds. Gently return to neutral position, then repeat the stretch on the other side. Complete one repetition on each side.

- **Levator Stretch** (SC2, page 153). Sit with good posture. Turn your head 45 degrees, then bring your nose down toward the same armpit until you feel a stretch on the back side of your neck on the opposite side. Keep the stretch pain free. Hold for forty-five to sixty seconds. Gently return to neutral position, then repeat the stretch on the other side. Complete one repetition on each side.

- **Plank Twists** (EC27, page 212). Starting in a standard plank position on the floor with your hands directly below your shoulders, your head in line with your body, your knees locked straight, and your hips in line with your spine. Hold for ten seconds. Start to shift your weight toward one hand; twist your spine until you are reaching up toward the ceiling. Hold for ten seconds. Rotate back down to the starting position and hold for ten seconds. Shift toward the other hand and twist to the other direction, holding for ten seconds. End in the starting position and rest. Complete five repetitions per set; perform one set.

- **Wall Angels** (EC14, page 199). Stand against a wall with your feet two feet away from the wall and your entire back—from tailbone to head, including the middle of your back—flat against the wall by drawing your abdominal muscles in. Lift your arms over your head with your elbows bent while keeping your entire arms and back flat against the wall. Begin to move your arms up and down in an arcing motion, moving only in the range in which you can keep your back flat against the wall. Complete ten repetitions per set; perform two sets.

- **Wall Push-ups** (EC15, page 200- done without the the Swiss ball). Place your hands directly on a wall slightly below the level of your shoulders. Extend your arms and gently squeeze your shoulder blades together and down toward your hips in a "V" position. Bend your elbows, allowing your upper body to move toward the wall as far as you comfortably can until you are in a push-up position. Push away from the wall, returning to the starting position. Complete ten repetitions per set; perform two sets.

Lumbar - On the Go!

- **Hamstring Stretch** (SL7, page 171). Lie on your back on the floor with both knees bent and feet flat on the floor. Place a towel or belt around one foot. Extend your leg until your knee is straight. Pull the strap toward your head, raising your leg up until you feel a stretch in the back of the leg. Hold for forty-five to sixty seconds. Repeat the stretch with the other leg. Perform one repetition with each leg.

- **Piriformis Stretch on Mat** (SL5, page 169). Lie on your back on the floor with your knees bent and your feet flat on the floor. Cross one leg over the other so that your ankle rests on the opposite knee. Hold the stretch for forty-five to sixty seconds. If no stretch is felt, begin to pull the opposite leg toward your chest until you feel a stretch, then hold it for forty-five to sixty seconds. Complete one repetition.

- **Up Crunches** (EL11, page 223). Lie on your back on the floor. Place a Swiss ball or folded pillow between your knees and gently squeeze. Bring your knees up to 90 degrees at your hips. Move your legs three inches toward your chest, engaging your upper abdominal muscles to "crunch" your knees toward your chest. Return your knees to the level of your hips and perform ten repetitions. Relax and place your feet on the floor to rest. Perform two sets.

- **Down Crunches** (EL12, page 224). Lie on your back on the floor. Place a Swiss ball or folded pillow under your knees and gently squeeze. Bring your knees up to 90 degrees at your hips. Slowly lower your legs toward the floor, moving two inches while keeping your back flat on the floor. Pull your knees back up to hip level. Complete ten repetitions, then relax and place your feet on the floor to rest. Perform two sets.

- **Froggies** (EL31, page 243) Start by sitting on the floor. Roll back onto your buttocks so that you are able to maintain your balance with your feet off the floor. Slowly lean your trunk back toward the floor while extending your feet out away from your body. Complete ten repetitions per set; perform two sets.

- **Bridge with Leg Extension** (EL21, 233). Lie on your back with your knees bent and your feet flat on the floor. Raise your hips off the floor, and extend one leg straight while keeping your hips level. Hold for five seconds. Place your foot back on the floor and extend the other leg while keeping your hips up in the air. Hold for five seconds. Place your foot back on the floor and lower your hips back to the starting position. Complete five repetitions per set; perform two sets.

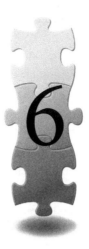

DMR Method Research

The DMR Method is based on research conducted since 2006 by the DMR Method research team. It began as a series of meetings between physical therapists, chiropractors, orthopedists, neurosurgeons, and radiologists whose goal was to learn how to work together better to improve patient care and outcomes. The DMR Method, which has since helped thousands of patients avoid spinal surgery and other invasive procedures, is the first integrated protocol of care combining the knowledge and skill of a wide range of healthcare professionals backed by research utilizing pre- and post-treatment MRIs and functional index scores (which track a person's ability to engage in normal physical activities). What follows is a summary of the DMR Method research conducted thus far, as well as a glimpse at current and future DMR Method research.

The Pilot DMR Method Clinical Case Study

Based upon initial outcomes after introducing the DMR Method to selected patients, an initial pilot DMR Method clinical case study was designed with the following goals:

- measure effectiveness of the method in treating disc herniations, degenerative disc disease, facet syndrome, and chronic neck and back pain using short- and long-term subjective, objective, and functional measures;

- identify patient lifestyle factors—physical, nutritional, and emotional— which may affect outcomes, and develop effective methods to address these factors;
- study changes in disc herniation position and size using recumbent, weight- bearing, and positional MRIs;
- study changes in degenerative disease, alignment, and stability of the spine using recumbent, weight-bearing, and positional MRI;
- use outcome data to further refine and improve the DMR Method procedures, protocols, and outcomes.

Conclusions

Twenty patients participated in the initial pilot DMR method clinical case study. Seventeen of the twenty completed the study with significant to marked improvements objectively, subjectively, and functionally. Most notable were the changes evidenced on many of the follow-up MRI evaluations when compared to initial, pre-DMR Method MRI evaluations. These follow-up MRIs showed shrinking and/or complete reabsorption of disc herniations diagnosed on the initial MRI evaluations.

Of the three patients who did not show significant improvement, one voluntarily left the program and subsequently had surgery with poor results. The other two patients experienced limited improvement within the eight-week period of treatment. In both cases, it was discovered in follow-up evaluations that neither had been consistent with self-care and rehab procedures. Following additional DMR Method patient education and rehabilitation, both patients attained excellent results.

Significant observations from the initial pilot DMR Method clinical case study include:

- the DMR Method is a highly effective way to treat herniated intervertebral discs as well as chronic back and neck pain;
- the DMR Method can significantly decrease the symptoms associated with the above conditions (back/neck/arm/leg pain, numbness and/or weakness);
- nineteen of the twenty initial case study participants (95 percent) experienced significant a decrease or resolution of their symptoms and an improvement in their ability to be physically active without symptoms (determined by attaining at least 30 percent improvement in functional index scores);

- patient satisfaction with the DMR Method was excellent.;
- the collaborative DMR Method evaluation and treatment process is a viable way to treat disc herniations;
- intervertebral disc herniations can partially or completely reabsorb;
- the larger the intervertebral disc herniation, the greater the potential for reabsorption;
- resolution and stabilization of a patient's condition is not solely reliant on the reabsorption of a herniated intervertebral disc; while partial or complete reabsorption was visualized in many of the follow-up MRIs, some cases with excellent clinical, subjective, and functional improvement showed no change in the size or position of a herniation on the follow-up MRIs.;
- the common factor in the two cases that didn't initially achieve excellent outcomes was their lack of participation in the rehabilitation component of the program;
- the rehabilitation component is essential to long-term success;
- although disc herniations can partially or completely reabsorb, there was no observable change in intervertebral disc hydration to the extent that was visualized on follow-up MRIs (except in two cases);
- when intervertebral disc herniations partially or completely reabsorb, it is unlikely that they reabsorb back into the body of the intervertebral disc. It appears that the herniation is reabsorbed into the surrounding interstitial fluid. This is based on the observation that there was no appreciable change in intervertebral disc thickness after large intervertebral disc herniations were shown to be completely reabsorbed on follow-up MRIs.

The First DMR Method Clinical Case Study (DMR1)

Based on the findings of the initial pilot DMR Method clinical case study, the DMR Method research team refined different components of the DMR Method and also established three distinct phases in the DMR Method treatment protocol; the relief, repair, and rehabilitation phases. They also developed specific patient education strategies to improve patient compliance and satisfaction. This formed the foundation for the first DMR Method clinical case study, a.k.a. the DMR1 Study.

Key developments based on the DMR1 study include:

- fully 96.4 percent of patients attained significant symptomatic and functional improvement when including data from lumbar and cervical cases (50% or greater improvement in functional index scores);

- recovery rates improved with the refinement of the DMR Method evaluation, treatment, and education protocols: patients averaged a 51.1 percent decrease in pain and disability as assessed by Oswestry Disability Questionnaire;

DMR Method Study
Hopkins Health & Wellness Center Physical Therapy
Case Studies

Acute Disc Herniation Case 1: Left lower back pain and S1 Radiculopathy

Pre-DMR Method MRI

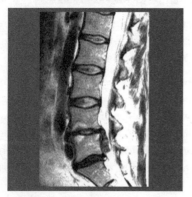

Post-DMR Method MRI

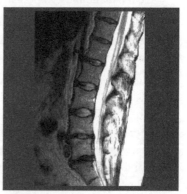

9-24-07: Large extruded caudally extending left posterolateral L4-5 disc herniation and large disc fragment behind the upper half of the L4 vertebral body. A second extruded high signal intensity disc herniation at L3-4 with left L3 nerve root impingement.

11-16-07: There has been significant interval change with marked regression of the disc herniation behind L3 and also marked regression of the disc herniation extruding caudally on the left behind L4.

2/1/15 Patient Update: continued symptom resolution. Continues with frequent self-care program. Functional capacity is excellent.

- disc herniations completely reabsorbed 100 percent of the time when patients began treatment within eight weeks of disc herniation occurrence, clearly suggesting that early intervention plays a significant role in recovery;

- long-term outcomes are excellent for patients who consistently follow the self-care protocols established during the DMR Method treatment progression;

DMR Method Study
Hopkins Health & Wellness Center Physical Therapy
Case Studies

Acute Disc Herniation Case 2: Lower back pain and Left L5 radiculopathy

Pre-DMR Method MRI

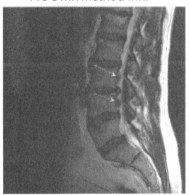

Post-DMR Method MRI

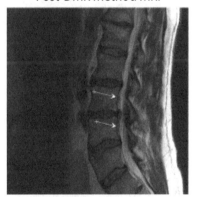

9-24-07: Large extruded caudally extending left posterolateral L4-5 disc herniation and large disc fragment behind the upper half of the L4 vertebral body. A second extruded high signal intensity disc herniation at L3-4 with left L3 nerve root impingement.

11-16-07: There has been significant interval change with marked regression of the disc herniation behind L3 and also marked regression of the disc herniation extruding caudally on the left behind L4.

2/1/15 Patient Update: continued symptom resolution. Continues with frequent self-care program. Functional capacity is excellent.

DMR Method Study
Hopkins Health & Wellness Center Physical Therapy
Case Studies

Acute Disc Herniation Case 3: Left lower back pain and S1 Radiculopathy

Pre-DMR Method MRI   Post-DMR Method MRI

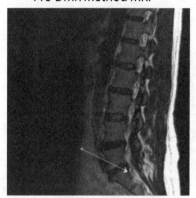   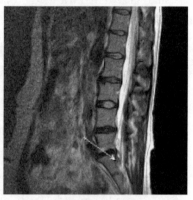

2-06-09: Moderate-sized caudally extruded left posterolateral disc herniation at L5-S1 with left S1 nerve root impingement as noted on the open upright MRI

4-01-09: Resorption of the moderate-sized, caudally extruded left posterolateral herniation at L5-S1 and resolution of related left S1 nerve root impingement since 02/06/09

2/1/15 Patient Update: continued symptom resolution. Continues with dialy DMR-Method self-care program. Continues to follow preventative restrictions. Functional capacity status is excellent and patient has resumed and maintained aggressive fitness training.

- a specific progression of joint manipulation was developed by the DMR Method chiropractic team called Integrated Progressive Manipulation (IPM);

- a specific protocol of manual muscle therapy was developed by the DMR Method research team called Dynamic Muscle Technique (DMT);

- A specific progression of standard traction (called DMR Method Progressive Traction) was developed by the DMR Method research team.

The DMR2 Clinical Case Study

The DMR Method research team began conducting the DMR2 clinical case study in 2011. DMR Method evaluation and treatment protocols had been further refined based on the findings of the pilot and DMR1 studies. One important refinement was the addition of the use of medical pain management protocols to assist in progressing difficult cases involving acute pain and inflammation.

Another key change based on the findings of the DMR1 Study concerned the time frame for follow-up MRIs performed on study participants. The spinal radiologists observed that many intervertebral disc herniations that were partially reabsorbed may have been in the process of healing and possibly would have shown more complete reabsorption if the follow-up MRI evaluation was performed later in the process. Consequently, the follow-up MRI evaluations in the DMR2 Clinical Case Study are taking place six months after the initial MRI evaluation.

The DMR2 Clinical Case Study was in process at the time this book was published; however, initial review of outcomes indicate a higher rate of disc herniation reabsorption and further improvement in pain and disability scores.

DMR Method Innovation

Currently, the DMR Method research team is developing a new piece of equipment called the DMR Lumbar Stabilizer, designed to help patients traction, stretch, and strengthen the lumbar spine. We expect this home-based self-care device to improve long-term outcomes by giving DMR Method patients a tool that decreases the need for clinical care.

To help quantify spinal dysfunction as well as help measure outcomes, the DMR Method research team is also developing a new diagnostic tool called proprioceptometry. If successful, it will offer doctors and therapists new insights into how spinal injuries and dysfunction affect the part of the nervous system responsible for giving the body its sense of position. It is our hope that measuring proprioception in the spine can provide an alternative way of objectively measuring spinal dysfunction and measuring improvement of spinal function with different forms of treatment.

Disc herniations and listhesis type spinal lesions treated nonsurgically; clinical correlations and observation via upright MRI

Peter L'Allier, DC*, Hopkins Health & Wellness Center

Abstract

Objective: Study the effects of a specific protocol (the DMR Advanced Protocol; see chapter 4) of physical therapy and chiropractic treatment on disc pathology and listhesis-type lesions both clinically and objectively via magnetic resonance imaging (MRI).

Methods: Twenty-three patients with spinal lesions were treated nonsurgically for eight to ten weeks with a specific regimen of treatment (the DMR Advanced Protocol). Objective data regarding the quantity and quality of spinal lesions were obtained through upright MRI study both before and after treatment so results could be compared to baseline data.

Results: Treatment produced significant changes in Oswestry Disability Index scores,, disc herniation size and resolve of neurologic compromise.

Conclusions: The nonsurgical, conservative DMR protocol of treatment provides equally effective treatment for disc herniations and discogenic neurologic compromise in a fraction of the time of traditional medical management and rehabilitation.

Study Type: Practice-based retrospective observational cohort of consecutive patients with lumbar disc herniation, disc bulge, or listhesis.

Key Words: lumbar disc herniation, neurologic compromise, DMR protocol, conservative treatment, magnetic resonance imaging, physical therapy.

*Clinician, Peter L'Allier, DC, Hopkins Health & Wellness Center, Hopkins, MN, USA

Corresponding Author: Pete L'Allier, PT@hopkinswellness.com

This study was supported by Hopkins Health & Wellness Center. Nothing of value was received from a commercial entity related to this manuscript.

Submit Reprint Requests to: Shannon Jones, Hopkins Health & Wellness Center, 15 8th Avenue N, Hopkins, MN 55343, tel. 952-933-5085, PT@hopkinswellness. com.

Introduction

Lumbar disc herniation is the most common musculoskeletal cause of low-back pain in patients under forty-five years of age.[6] Treatment for lumbar disc herniation has been a topic of research for nearly fifty years. Surgeries for disc herniation are the most common surgery performed on the spine.16 Current data suggests residual back pain in 74 percent of lumbar disc herniation surgery patients, 12 percent of who required repeat surgery.[24] With the high rate of failed surgery, current research often focuses on the use of conservative treatment in the care of patients with lumbar disc herniation.

With the greater availability of advanced imaging, numerous studies have observed the natural history of herniations. Spontaneous reabsorption is now a well-documented part of the natural clinical progression of this condition.[1-11,19-21,23] It is now well accepted that, given time and conservative treatment, disc herniations will reduce in size. Conservative care has been demonstrated to be more cost effective and equally as effective as surgery in long-term studies.[2,6,8,16,21] Most research suggests an average treatment time of thirty-four to forty-three weeks is sufficient to treat disc herniations conservatively.[2,4-6,9,11,18,23] However, "conservative treatment" is not uniformly defined. The majority of studies researching conservative treatment of lumbar disc herniations utilize such medical procedures as epidural steroid injections, epidural blocks, nerve blocks, analgesics, medications. and bed rest.[2,3,6,8,11,16,21,23] Few studies have investigated lumbar disc herniations without the use of medical intervention.

In the current study, treatment includes a specific protocol of conservative treatment called the DMR protocol. This study seeks to observe and analyze the effects of the DMR protocol of conservative treatment in the management of lumbar disc herniations, disc bulges, and listhesis type lesions.

Materials and Methods

Twenty-three consecutive patients presenting with low-back pain or leg pain who were treated for disc herniation or lumbar listhesis were selected for the study. These patients each completed paperwork, pre- and post-Oswestry Disability Questionnaires, and two MRI studies. Of the study participants, 60 percent were male and 40 percent were female, with an average overall age of fifty-two. Of these twenty-three patients, 24 percent presented within eight weeks of onset of symptoms and were considered still in the acute phase of injury. The median age of those patients admitted in the acute phase was 47.5, while the median age of those presenting with chronic low-back pain was 54.

Conservative treatment of the twenty-three patients included a specific protocol of physical therapy and chiropractic treatment called the DMR Method protocol. This nonsurgical treatment protocol is a progressive process of manual therapy, specific spinal manipulation, adjunctive therapies, mechanical spinal traction, and an extensive personalized rehabilitative process. The rehabilitative process includes posture, ergonomics, and body mechanics education; stretching and flexibility techniques; and a exercise program that focuses on strength, stability, and spinal balance. Nutritional supplements were also provided to assist soft-tissue healing. Patients were seen in-office for twenty to twenty-four visits over an eight-to-ten-week period. The frequency of care was gradually reduced from three times per week to two.

The twenty-three study participants completed an Oswestry Disability Index Questionnaire to evaluate function and disability due to pain prior to treatment (scored 0 to 100, with a greater score representing a greater degree of disability). The questionnaire was again completed following the completion of eight to ten weeks of conservative treatment. Change in individual scores was calculated as:

([initial score - final score]/initial score) x 100 = percent improvement

Additionally, t-test statistical analysis was performed to evaluate the significance of the change in scores.

MRI studies were obtained prior to treatment and immediately following treatment. MRI scans were performed on a 0.75T upright scanner. T2 upright neutral, flexion, and extension sagittal images, T1 neutral sagittal and T2-weighted axial images were obtained during each evaluation. Both MRI studies were evaluated by the same radiologist, acting as an independent investigator. The radiologist was to report the presence of any disc bulges, herniations, or listhesis-type lesions and quantify the lesions. Herniations were to be classified as protrusions or extrusions. Listhesis-type lesions were evaluated for dynamic quality on sagittal flexion and extension scans. Data and change in quality and quantity of lesions was recorded and evaluated with t-test analysis. The change in size of lesions was defined as:

(1-[lesion size on later scan/lesion size on initial scan]) x 100 = percent improvement

Results

Decreases in pain and disability were found in 100 percent of patients. Patients averaged a 51.1 percent decrease in pain and disability as assessed by

Oswestry Disability Questionnaire. The average initial score decreased from 35 percent to 16.7 percent. This difference was statistically significant, with a p-value of 1.1E-5. Further, 43 percent of patients experienced a decrease in pain and disability greater than 50 percent. The majority of patients (82 percent) achieved an increase in function greater than 25 percent. The greatest changes in pain and disability (66 percent) were noted in those patients presenting in an acute phase of less than eight weeks duration. Those presenting with chronic low-back pain experienced, on average, a decrease of 43.2 percent in pain and disability, which is still significant.

The greatest decrease in pain and disability was noted in those patients presenting in the age group of fifty to fifty-nine. On average, this group experienced a decrease in pain and disability of 60.1 percent. The age group experiencing the least reduction in symptoms and disability were those in the seventy to seventy-nine age group. This is consistent with the pathophysiology of this condition as the degree of disc hydration, and therefore the body's ability to reabsorb, greatly decreases with age.

This study also showed a correlation between gender and degree of functional improvement. Female patients experienced an average 66.6 percent decrease in pain and disability; in comparison, male patients only experienced a 39.2 percent decrease, a statistically significant difference with p-value of 0.019. The women (average age of 50.6) were slightly younger than the men (average age of 54.3). On average, the women completed the protocol in eleven weeks, while the men completed treatment in 10.6 weeks. Neither the differences in age or duration of treatment are statistically significant.

The MRI data revealed a statistically significant difference in the change of both disc herniation and listhesis-type lesion size. The greatest changes in disc herniation size were noted among those presenting in the acute stage (57.1 percent) of injury and women (44 percent), despite the greater number of herniations in men and those presenting with chronic conditions. The average degree of change in herniation size was 42.1 percent among those experiencing a change. Reabsorption occurred in 100 percent of the disc herniations treated within eight weeks of occurrence. Similar to previous studies, the greatest degree of change was noted in larger lesions. Herniations measuring greater than 8mm decreased by an average 76 percent over the course of the eight to ten weeks of treatment.

In addition to the resolution or modification of lesions, neurologic compromise was also evaluated. The treatment utilized in this study produced statistically significant resolution of neurologic compromise, p-value 0.021, via MRI. Overall, 60 percent of those experiencing reduction were women and 60 percent presented in the acute phase of injury.

A correlation between resolution of neurologic compromise and restored function was quite high, with a p-value of 0.0093. Those who experienced a reduction of demonstrable neurologic compromise had an average change in Oswestry Disability Index of 79.1 percent. This is strikingly different from the average 33.8 percent change in Oswestry scores experienced by those without resolution of neurologic compromise.

Discussion

Lumbar lesions such as disc herniations, disc bulges, and listhesis are common occurrences. Herniations are reported to naturally occur in 31 to 33 percent of an asymptomatic population.[6,17] The natural history of lumbar disc herniations is to spontaneously regress.[1-11,19-21,23] Though the mechanism is not understood completely, research points to the involvement of macrophages in phagocytosis of discal remnants.[8,10,19-20,23] This process involves the combination of inflammation and neovascularization for phagocytosis.[10]

The use of MRI may provide some clinical indications as to the likelihood of herniations to reabsorb. The herniated disc material is more likely to be reabsorbed if it has violated the posterior longitudinal ligament as the likelihood of neovascularization is greater.[2,11,23] In addition to disruption of the PLL, the signal of the disc on a T2 weighted scan may be indicative of reabsorption. The greater the intensity of T2 signal, the more likely a disc herniation is to reabsorb.[8,11] However, the natural healing process of the disc herniation via reabsorption will cause an increase in degenerative disc disease at the level of herniation.[1,19,22] Thus the greater the initial T2 signal, the greater the level of dehydration and resulting reabsorption of disc material. Finally, the size of the lesion itself may be an indication as to the degree of reabsorption. Numerous studies have demonstrated that the larger the size of the herniation, the greater the degree of reabsorption.[2,4-5,10-11]

Similar results were demonstrated in this study, as 60 percent of those herniations measuring greater than 8mm had an average 76 percent decrease in size over the course of treatment. Overall, a statistically significant difference was found in regards to the decrease in size of disc herniations following treatment. Furthermore, patients enrolled in treatment experienced an average 23.8 percent decrease in the quantity of neurologic compromise as noted on MRI.

With the increased knowledge of the natural history of disc herniations, more research has been done on the conservative treatment of such conditions. Conservative care, though shown to be cost effective, is not well defined.[2,6,8,16,21] Spinal steroid injections are one of the most common conservative care interventions for pain and inflammation control in the research of patients with lumbar disc herniations.[2-3,6,8,11,16,21] The efficacy of steroid injections, however, has been demonstrated to be limited to inflammation and pain reduction as it does not aid the reabsorption of disc material.[11] Memmo, et al., reported that 32 percent of patients who received surgery for lumbar discectomy had previously received an injection.[16]

Very little research exists on the nonmedical treatment of disc pathology. Favorable results have been reported with treatment utilizing physical therapy and/or chiropractic manipulations.[9,19,22] Though both medical and nonmedical treatments report positive results, the average treatment time for nonmedical interventions is drastically less.[2,4-6,9,11,18,22,24] The average study of nonmedical treatment (chiropractic or physical therapy) consisted of 3.5 weeks of care, whereas the average medical conservative care plan studied averaged thirty-nine to sixty-five weeks. This significant difference in treatment duration may have greater social implications in terms of time away from work caused by pain or decreased function.

In the current study, patients were prescribed eight to ten weeks of conservative treatment, including the DMR protocol of physical therapy and chiropractic treatment. Fully 78 percent of patients completed the prescribed treatment plan and MRI scans within the allotted time; however, five patients took longer than eleven weeks to complete treatment. All patients saw a decrease in clinical symptoms and an increase in function, as determined by Oswestry Disability Questionnaire. On average, those patients that completed the program within ten weeks saw a decrease in Oswestry Scores of 46.7 percent, which is slightly lower than the average 67.1 percent decrease seen by those who took longer than eleven weeks to complete the treatment plan. Of those patients receiving treatment longer than ten weeks, 60 percent were chronic cases. Such data suggests that perhaps a treatment period of greater than ten weeks may be beneficial to the treatment of chronic conditions. The data also supports previous findings that nonmedical treatments can be equally effective while requiring much less time.

Studies have consistently shown the spontaneous reabsorption of disc herniations in 63 to 95 percent of patients.[1,11,23] Studies have shown continued reabsorption over time, up to 95 percent at seven years post injury. 1 In addition, it is reported that 63 to 78 percent of all herniated discs will reduce in size to some degree over the course of a few years.[3,5-6,11,21] Reabsorption of more than 50 percent of disc herniation size may be seen in 48 to 50 percent of people with lumbar disc herniations.[5,23] The greatest results are demonstrated by larger initial herniations.[8,11] The resolution of disc bulges, however, is much less likely with conservative treatment. Bush K, et al., demonstrated that only 26 percent of disc bulges resolved with conservative treatment.[3]

The current study revealed a statistically significant difference in the size of herniations following treatment, with a p-value of 0.05. Of those patients, 57.1 percent presenting within the acute stage of injury saw reduction of 50 percent or more of the herniation size of one or more herniations within the treatment time of two months. These results are slightly better than those of previous studies despite the great variation in the duration of treatment in those studies. With follow-up MRI studies being obtained, on average, ten weeks following initial presentation, the duration of the current study was roughly 12 to 20 percent of the average treatment time of other medical studies. It is predicted that follow-up studies performed closer to twelve to eighteen months following initial presentation would demonstrate greater results.

In addition to the statistically significant reabsorption of disc herniations, the resolution of neurologic compromise in patients was also statistically significant in this study, with a p-value of 0.021. Patients experienced an average 23.81 percent reduction in neurologic compromise demonstrated via MRI. Further, 42.86 percent of patients experienced a complete resolution of neurologic compromise at one or more spinal levels following the ten-week nonmedical treatment. Women and those presenting with acute conditions were more likely to experience resolution of neurologic compromise (60 percent).

Though the presence of neurologic compromise is not necessarily indicative of pain, the change in Oswestry scores for those experiencing a reduction in neurologic compromise was 79.1 percent, as compared to the 33.8 percent who experienced no change in neurologic compromise. This statistically significant difference, with p-value of 0.0093, also correlates with the resolution of disc herniations. A statistically significant difference, p-value 0.005, was apparent between the degree of resolution of herniations among those experiencing resolution of neurologic compromise and those who did not. These significant correlations support the idea that herniations causing neurologic compromise are indeed the source of much pain and functional disability. It also suggests that resolution of neural pressure and irritation may significantly improve function and reduce pain.

Similar to previous studies, the resolution of disc bulges was unimpressive. In the ten-week treatment, 22.2 percent of patients with disc bulges experienced resolution of their bulge. This is not a significant difference (p-value 0.17). In addition, of those patients presenting with listhesis-type lesions, only 15.8 percent experienced resolution of the lesion. This is not statistically significant (p-value 0.1). All of the patients experiencing resolution of a disc bulge or listhesis presented with chronic low-back pain.

The conservative care of disc herniations has proved to be highly effective clinically. Studies have reported subjective improvements from 65 to 96 percent with various screening tools.[1,2,6,8,11,18] For the purpose of this study, the Oswestry Disability Index Questionnaire was used to evaluate pain and functional disability because of its high degree of responsiveness.[13] The Oswestry Disability Questionnaire is scored 0 to 100 percent (the greater the score, the greater the degree of functional disability). Unlu Z, et al., demonstrated the average base line Oswestry Score for patients with one or more disc herniations as being 19.1 percent.[9] Following treatment with one physical therapy modality, Unlu demonstrated a decrease in Oswestry score to an average 14.6 percent, an average change of 23.56 percent.[9]

The results of the current study demonstrated far greater clinical improvement than the aforementioned study. The current study resulted in 100 percent of patients seeing some degree of increase in function. The average initial Oswestry score upon presentation was 35 percent disability. The average Oswestry score following the treatment protocol was 16.7 percent— an average 51.1 percent decrease in functional disability, with p-value of 1.12E-5. This change is over two times of that demonstrated by Unlu utilizing one-physical therapy modality.[9]

The greatest restoration of functional ability was noted among those patients who presented in the acute phase. These patients saw a 66 percent increase in function within ten weeks of treatment. 100 percent of the patients presenting for treatment in the acute phase (within eight weeks of disc herniation occurrence) showed disc herniation reabsorption on post-treatment MRI evaluations. Still significant increases of an average 43.2 percent were seen in those who presented with chronic low-back conditions of more than two months in duration. Further, 43 percent of the patients in the study obtained greater than a 50 percent increase in function following ten weeks of treatment. These significant improvements in such a short duration of treatment suggest the high degree of efficacy of nonmedical treatment of disc pathology and listhesis lesions, and that early intervention can improve outcomes..

Complications of this study, like any study, will limit the relevance of conclusions. One complication that arose in this study was the inconsistency of treatment. While the majority of patients completed treatment in the recommended time, a few outliers took longer to complete treatment. In addition, while all patients completed the same protocol, there were some variations within the protocol regarding stretches, exercises, etc. that may have been specifically tailored to the patient's needs. A follow-up study that would control these areas of variability may provide more valid conclusions.

Conclusions

On average, patients experienced a 50.1 percent increase in function within ten weeks of treatment. Disc herniation reabsorption can be improved with treatment. The size of the herniation as well as the time elapsed from disc herniation occurrence and treatment can have an influence on reabsorption rates. The best results were obtained by those presenting within eight weeks of injury, women, and those between the ages of fifty to fifty-nine. Strong correlations exist between the presence of neurologic compromise, functional disability, and pain. Conservative, nonsurgical treatment with the DMR protocol may be highly effective in the treatment of disc herniations and neurologic compromise caused by such pathology. Further, resolution of disc herniations and neurologic compromise with this nonsurgical treatment may be possible to achieve in far less time than with accepted medical interventions.

Acknowledgements

The authors would like to thank William J. Mullin, M.D., Spine Radiologist; Timothy Mick, DC F.I.C.C., D.A.B.C.R.; and Thomas J. Gilbert, M.D., M.P.P. at The Center for Diagnostic Imaging for their assistance in interpretation of the Magnetic Resonance Imaging studies and assisting in selection of imaging sequences. We would also like to thank Jannel P. Kammerer, MPT for helping to develop and administer the initial physical therapy treatment protocol. Finally, we would like to thank the clinical staff of Hopkins Health & Wellness Center for providing excellent healthcare services to all patients in the study. A special thank you to Stephanie E. Musselman, DC, MS, DACB for her hard work in organizing all the case study data and statistical analysis. Without her help and research expertise, this study would not have been possible.

References

1. Masui T, et al. Natural history of patients with lumbar disc herniation observed by magnetic resonance imaging for a minimum of seven years. J Spinal Disord Tech 2005;18:121-126.
2. Ito T, Takano Y, Yuasa N. Types of lumbar herniated disc and clinical course. Spine 2001;26(6):648-651.
3. Bush K, Cowan N, Katz D, Gishen P. The natural history of sciatica associated with disc pathology: a prospective study with clinical and independent radiologic follow-up. Spine 1992;17(10):1205-1212.

4. Yukawa, et al. Serial Magnetic Resonance Imaging follow-up study of lumbar disc herniation conservatively treated for average 30 months: relation between reduction of herniation and degeneration of disc. J of Spinal Disord 1996;9(3):251-256.

5. Bozzao A, et al. Lumbar disc herniation: MR imaging assessment of natural history in patients treated without surgery. Radiology 1992;185:135-141.

6. Memmo P, Nadler S, Malanga G. Lumbar disc herniations: a review of surgical and nonsurgical indications and outcomes. J of Back and Msk Rehab 2000;14:79-88.

7. Saal J, Saal J, Herzog R. The natural history of lumbar intervertebral disc extrusions treated non-opperatively. Spine 1990;15:683-686.

8. Saal J, Saal J. Lumbar disc extrusions with radiculopathy: natural history of resolution with non-opperative management. Spine 2003;3:83S.

9. Unlu Z, Tascl S, Tarhan S, Pabuscu Y, Islak S. Comparison of three Physical Therapy modalities for acute pain in lumbar disc herniation measured by clinical evaluation and magnetic resonance imaging. JMPT 2008;31(3):191-198.

10. Autio R, et al. Determinants of spontaneous reabsorption of intervertebral disc herniations. Spine 2006;31(11):1247-1252.

11. Buttermann G. Lumbar disc herniation regression after successful epidural steroid injection. J of Spinal Disord &Tech 2002;15(6):469-476.

12. Khorsan R, Coulter I, Hawk C, Goertz Choate C. Measures in Chiropractic Research: Choosing patient-based outcome assessments. JMPT 2008;31(5):355-375.

13. Ferrari, R. Responsiveness of the Short-Form 36 and Oswestry Disability Questionnaire in chronic nonspecific low-back and lower-limb pain treated with customized foot orthotics. JMPT 2007;30(6):456-458.

14. Cooley J, Danielson C, Schultz G, Hall T. Posterior disk displacement: morphologic assessment and measurement reliability – lumbar spine. JMPT 2001;24(5):317-326.

15. Carragee E, Han M, Suen P, Kim D. Clinical outcomes after lumbar discectomy for sciatica: the effects of fragment type anular competence. J Bone & Joint Surgery 2003;85:102-108.

16. Daffner S, Hymanson H, Wang J. Cost and utilization of conservative management of lumbar disc herniation in patients undergoing surgical discectomy. Spine 2008;8:94S.

17. Borenstein D, et al. The value of magnetic resonance imaging of the lumbar spine to predict low-back pain in asymptomatic subjects. J Bone & Joint Surgery 2001;83:1306-1311.

18. Murphy D, Hurwitz E, McGovern E. A nonsurgical approach to the management of patients with lumbar radiculopathy secondary to disc herniation: a prospective observational cohort study with long-term follow-up. Spine 2008;8:161S.

19. Iwabuchi S, et al. Low intensity pulsed ultrasound enhances herniated disc reabsorption in a rat culture. Spine 2005;5:114S.

20. Tsuru M, et al. Spontaneous remission of intervertebral disk hernia and responses of surrounding macrophages. Spine 2003;3:82-83S.

21. Saal JS, Saal JA. Lumbar Stabilizing exercises for the nonoperative treatment of disc lesions. California Medical Association. 432.

22. Santilli V, Beghi E, Finucci S. Chiropractic manipulation in the treatment of acute back pain and sciatica with disc protrusion: a randomized double-blinded clinical trial of active and simulated spinal manipulations. Spine 2006;6:131-137.

23. Borota L, Jonasson P, Agolli A. Spontaneous reabsorption of intradural lumbar disc fragments. Spine 2008;8:397-403.

24. Postacchini F. Lumbar disc herniation: a new equilibrium is needed between nonoperative and operative treatment. Spine 2001;26(6):601.

DMR Method ®
Clinical Case Studies

DMR Method™ Case Study

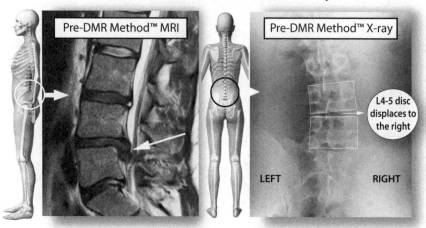

Pre-DMR Method™ MRI

Pre-DMR Method™ X-ray

L4-5 disc displaces to the right

LEFT   RIGHT

Lumbar Disc Herniation

Andrew was diagnosed with a herniated disc between L4 and L5. It caused local back pain that radiated down his right leg into his calf, which made it difficult for him to stand for long periods of time while he saw patients. He had been trying medical management and rehab therapy for nine months without success.

DIAGNOSIS

An MRI confirmed an L4-5 disc herniation causing irritation to the nerves going into Andrew's right leg (see left photo above). DMR Method Evaluation, including X-rays, revealed immobility and misalignment of the joints in the lower lumbar spine and pelvis that forced the L4-5 disc to herniate to the right side (see right photo above). Note: Surgery would remove the herniation, but do nothing to fix the imbalance in the spine that led to the disc herniation.

TREATMENT

Andrew completed the Chronic Lumbar DMR Protocol with a focus on restoring mobility, alignment and stability to the lower lumbar spine and pelvis.

OUTCOME

Andrew's symptoms quickly resolved and he was able to resume normal physical activities at home and at work. 5 year follow-up revealed no recurrence of disc herniation. He continues with a self-care stretching program and periodic DMR Method maintenance care.

DMR Method™ Case Study

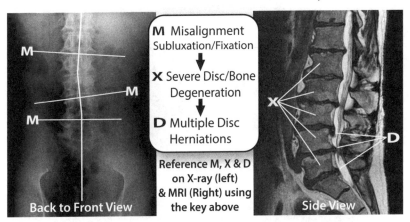

M Misalignment
Subluxation/Fixation

↓

X Severe Disc/Bone
Degeneration

↓

D Multiple Disc
Herniations

Reference M, X & D
on X-ray (left)
& MRI (Right) using
the key above

Back to Front View

Side View

Multiple Severe Disc Herniations & Degeneration Lumbar Spine

Over the course of seven years, Bruce developed lower back pain that increasingly radiated down his left leg into his foot and eventually became disabling. Medical pain management was unsuccessful and he was referred for an MRI. His doctor subsequently recommended back surgery. Before proceeding with surgery, Bruce decided to have a DMR Method consult based on the recommendation of a friend.

DIAGNOSIS

An MRI done on 12/10/09 revealed a large extruded left-sided disc herniation at L3-L4 causing severe compression of the L4 nerve root. Also noted were disc herniations with nerve compression at L4-5 and L5-S1. DMR Method Evaluation revealed severe fixation and misalignment/subluxation of the lumbar spine with muscle spasm and ligamentous restriction (see X-ray (left) and MRI (right) above).

TREATMENT

DMR Method Chronic Protocol for multiple disc herniations, with focus on phase 1 to phase 3 Integrated Dynamic Mobilization (IDM) due to severity of fixation/misalignment/subluxation of the spine.

OUTCOME

Complete resolution of back and leg symptoms. Return to normal physical activities including riding his motorcycle and snowmobiling. His five-year follow-up confirmed continued symptom resolution, and he continues with preventative care.

DMR Method™ Case Study

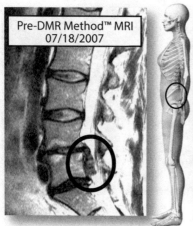
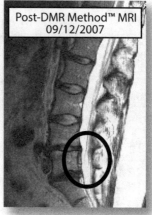

Pre-DMR Method™ MRI
07/18/2007

Post-DMR Method™ MRI
09/12/2007

Severe Disc Herniation Lumbar Spine

Amy was loading her washing machine when she bent over to pick up a laundry basket. She felt something "go out" in her lower back and experienced an intense pain that began radiating down her left leg. Her leg pain soon progressed to numbness and weakness and she began to have difficulty walking. Based on MRI findings, medical radiologists recommended emergency surgery.

DIAGNOSIS

The MRI confirmed a severe extruded disc herniation at L4-5, causing nerve compression. DMR Method Evaluation revealed severe misalignment and immobility in the lower lumbar spine and pelvis, with severe muscle spasm and inflammation.

TREATMENT

Due to the severity of Amy's condition, her case was closely monitored. Her treatment following the completion of the Acute Lumbar DMR Protocol was focused on oscillating decompression traction, cold laser therapy and Integrated Progressive Mobilization (IPM).

OUTCOME

Amy experienced a resolution of all symptoms without needing surgery. Her extruded disc was entirely reabsorbed and she has been able to resume normal daily activities without pain. After seven years, Amy reports continued symptoms resolution and normal physical abilities.

NOTE: Amy was the very first DMR Method patient!

DMR Method™ Case Study

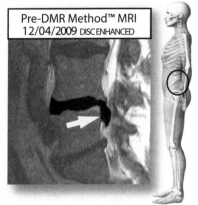

Pre-DMR Method™ MRI
12/04/2009 DISC ENHANCED

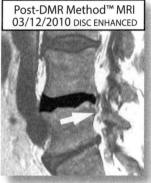

Post-DMR Method™ MRI
03/12/2010 DISC ENHANCED

L4 Disc Herniation Lumbar Spine

Joe developed a disc herniation in the lower lumbar spine and was referred by his doctor for orthopedic spine surgery. After a difficult recovery, his painful leg symptoms were gone but his back still didn't feel normal. While bending and lifting, he re-herniated the same disc; in addition to lower back pain, he developed disabling left leg pain. Instead of a second surgery, he decided to try the DMR Method.

DIAGNOSIS

MRI confirmed a large L4-5 extruded disc herniation causing left L5 nerve root compression. DMR Method Evaluation revealed misalignment/subluxation of lumbar spine and pelvis. Also noted were severe immobility, muscle spasm and ligament contracture.

TREATMENT

Joe completed the Acute Lumbar DMR Method Protocol, including restrictions, self-care instructions, a supportive nutrition program, Integrated Progressive Mobilization (IPM) and Dynamic Muscle Technique (DMT) to restore mobility, alignment and stability. He progressed to a self-care exercise and stretching program.

OUTCOME

Resolution of all symptoms, restored functional abilities and restored mobility, alignment and stability. A follow-up MRI revealed complete reabsorption of L4-5 disc herniation (see enhanced pre- and post-MRI images above). After four years, Joe reports continued symptom resolution and normal physical abilities.

DMR Method™ Case Study

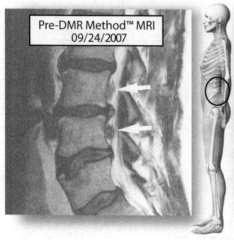

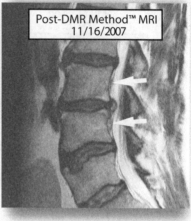

Multiple Disc Herniations Lumbar Spine

John developed severe debilitating lower back pain after lifting improperly. His pain continued for weeks and worsened after doing housework, radiating down his left leg. He couldn't stand without leaning forward and his leg felt weak and unstable.

DIAGNOSIS

An MRI scan revealed two large herniations between L4-5 and L3-4 in the lumbar spine causing left-sided nerve root impingement. DMR Method Evaluation revealed severe spinal immobility in the lumbar spine and pelvis, muscle and ligament remodeling and lower back and pelvic misalignment, causing excessive pressure on the lower lumbar discs.

TREATMENT

Acute Lumbar DMR Protocol for multiple herninations that included a lumbar support belt and strict limitations on physical activities to prevent aggravation or re-injury.

OUTCOME

Complete resolution of back and leg symptoms and a return to normal physical activity. A follow-up MRI eight weeks after the initial MRI revealed reabsorption of L4-5 and L3-4 disc herniations. His seven-year follow-up confirmed continued symptom resolution and normal to enhanced physical abilities.

DMR Method™ Case Study

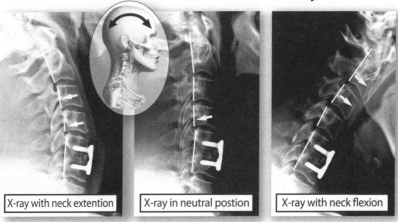

X-ray with neck extention | X-ray in neutral postion | X-ray with neck flexion

Neck and Arm Pain
Before and After Neck Fusion Surgery

Kevin had neck fusion surgery in November 2012. Following the surgery, he continued to have severe neck pain and stiffness. He also developed severe headaches and experienced pain in his arms that steadily escalated. After eight months with no improvement he was told he needed another surgery to fuse more of his neck. He opted to try the DMR Method™ instead.

DIAGNOSIS

X-ray evaluation revealed stable appliance fusion of C5-C6, but unstable motion of the vertebrae above the fusion (see x-rays above). DMR Method Evaluation revealed severe fixation/subluxation of the upper neck and upper thoracic spine with reactive muscle spasm and greater occipital nerve irritation (causing headaches), and brachial plexus nerve irritation (causing arm symptoms).

TREATMENT

Post-operative Cervical DMR Protocol with a contraindication to any mobilization of the surgically fused C5-C6 segment.

OUTCOME

Kevin avoided a second neck surgery. All of his symptoms—neck pain and stiffness, headaches and arm symptoms—were resolved. Due to the surgical fusion in his neck, he was educated about and advised to consistently follow home care and proactive DMR maintenance care.

DMR Method™ Case Study

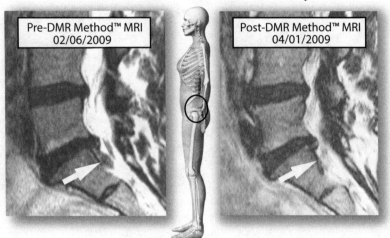

Pre-DMR Method™ MRI
02/06/2009

Post-DMR Method™ MRI
04/01/2009

Moderate Disc Herniation Lumbar Spine

Laura, who has a history of rheumatoid arthritis, was in an exercise class when she felt her back give out. The pain worsened over the next few hours and began causing numbness and weakness in her left leg. She couldn't bear weight on her left leg and couldn't sit, stand or walk without severe lower back and leg pain.

DIAGNOSIS

An MRI scan revealed a moderate left-sided L5-S1 disc herniation with nerve root compression. DMR Method Evaluation revealed severe immobility and misalignment of the lower lumbar spine and pelvis, plus muscle spasm, swelling, and remodeling/constriction of the muscles and ligaments in the lower lumbar spine and pelvis.

TREATMENT

Acute Lumbar DMR Protocol. Laura was also referred for a lumbar epidural injection to decrease acute pain and inflammation.

OUTCOME

Laura attained complete resolution of back and leg symptoms and returned to aggressive fitness activities. A follow-up MRI eight weeks after her initial MRI revealed complete reabsorption of the disc herniation. Her five-year follow-up revealed continued symptom resolution. Her arthritis-related back pain has been managed with stretching and periodic care. She maintains a very active lifestyle and manages her rheumatoid arthritis well.

DMR Method™ Case Study

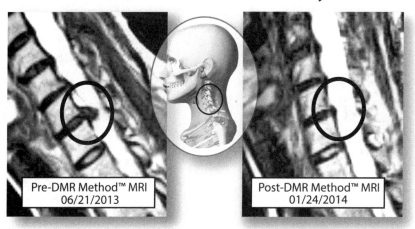

| Pre-DMR Method™ MRI | Post-DMR Method™ MRI |
| 06/21/2013 | 01/24/2014 |

Disc Herniation Cervical Spine

Sarah developed severe upper back pain after sleeping the wrong way on a hotel pillow. The pain progressed into her neck; over the next few days she began experiencing severe/constant tingling in her right hand. She had a difficult time sleeping because the pain and numbness worsened when she laid down.

DIAGNOSIS

An MRI scan on 6/21/13 revealed a severe C6-C7 disc herniation causing compression of the right C7 nerve. DMR Method Evaluation revealed severe fixation/subluxation and degeneration in the lower cervical and upper thoracic spine. Sarah also experienced extensive muscle spasm as well as ligament and joint capsule restriction.

TREATMENT

Acute Cervical DMR Method protocol with medical pain management, including epidural steroid injection to decrease pain and inflammation so Sarah could proceed with the DMR Method Protocol. One of the keys to her progression was the combination of Oscilating Decompression Traction (ODT) and Dynamic Muscle Technique (DMT).

OUTCOME

Sarah's neck, upper back and arm symptoms were completely resolved. A follow-up MRI on 1/24/14 revealed a marked reabsorption of the C6-C7 disc herniation (see enhanced pre- and post-MRI images above). She has resumed normal physical activity, including aggressive fitness training.

DMR Method™ Case Study

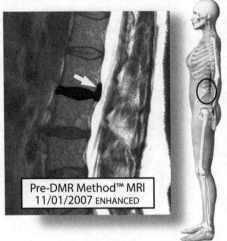

Pre-DMR Method™ MRI
11/01/2007 ENHANCED

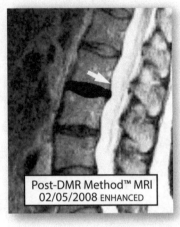

Post-DMR Method™ MRI
02/05/2008 ENHANCED

Lumbar Disc Herniation with Back Pain

Sandra developed acute severe lower back pain after bending forward to lift a very light object. After failing to improve with standard physical therapy and chiropractic treatment, she had an MRI scan done and came in for a DMR Method Evaluation.

DIAGNOSIS

The MRI scan confirmed a large 14mm x 4mm L2-3 disc herniation that extruded outward and upward (see image above). DMR Method Evaluation revealed joint immobility and misalignment/subluxation in the lumbar spine. Muscle imbalance and spasm was indicative of a structural condition that had been developing over a long period of time.

TREATMENT

Because of the new disc herniation, Sandra first completed the acute lumbar DMR Method Protocol with a focus on Integrated Progressive Mobilization (IPM). As her condition improved, her chiropractors and physical therapists transitioned her to a care program that focused on the correction of the long-term joint and muscle imbalance that was the true underlying cause of the new disc herniation.

OUTCOME

Sandra's back and leg pain resolved. A follow-up MRI showed a marked regression of the L2-3 disc herniation with 3mm x 3mm residual. Her six-year follow-up confirmed continued symptom resolution.

DMR Method™ Case Study

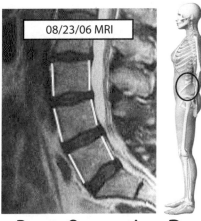

08/23/06 MRI

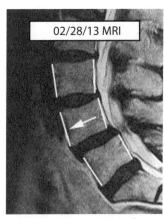

02/28/13 MRI

Post-Operative Degeneration and Slippage of Spine (Spondylolisthesis)

Sally had surgery on her lower back in 2006 (L4-5 laminectomy). She had recurrent incidental back pain post-surgery, but in 2012 her back pain and right leg pain became constant and severe; she couldn't walk without pain. Her doctor recommended injections and surgery. She was referred by a friend for a DMR Method consult.

DIAGNOSIS

A lumbar MRI done on 2/28/13 revealed post-operative forward slippage of the L4 vertabra with advanced joint degeneration and compression of the nerves in the lumbar spine. DMR Method Evaluation revealed severe restricted motion and compression of the lumbar spine with severe distortion and misalignment causing muscle, ligament, and joint capsule distortion.

TREATMENT

Chronic Lumbar DMR Protocol with a focus on joint mobilization, Decompression, and Progressive Muscle Technique.

OUTCOME

Due to the severity of her condition and her post-operative challenges, Sally's DMR Method progression was more gradual. In time, however, her symptoms resolved and she can now walk and be active without pain, which prevented the need for a second, more invasive back surgery. She prevents recurrence and maintains her pain-free lifestyle with stabilization exercises and periodic preventative care.

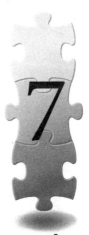

Frequently Asked Questions

What does DMR stand for?

Diagnose, Manage and Rehabilitate. The team of healthcare providers responsible for developing the DMR Method identified those three elements as essential for effective treatment. They then developed protocols for the three phases of recovery (relief, repair, and rehabilitation) and the three goals of treatment (mobility, alignment, and stability).

What exactly is the DMR Method treatment program?

The DMR Method is a specific course of evaluation and treatment based on years of clinical case study research utilizing pre- and post-treatment MRI scans and functional index scores (which track a person's ability to engage in normal physical activities). Evaluation and treatment is provided by a team of healthcare providers that may include physical therapists, chiropractors, and allied medical providers. Once the primary cause of a condition has been identified, treatment progresses through three phases: relief, repair, and rehabilitation. The primary goal of treatment is to decrease symptoms rapidly and improve the underlying cause of the condition by restoring mobility, alignment, and stability to the spine. After completing the DMR Method treatment program, the patient is given an after-care program to independently support and stabilize their recovery. For a more detailed description of the DMR Method evaluation and treatment program, please refer to chapters 3 and 4 in this book.

How is the DMR Method different than other nonsurgical spinal rehab programs?

There is no other spinal rehab program like the DMR Method. The DMR Method is a team effort between physical therapists, chiropractors, and allied medical doctors. It is a unique process of evaluation and treatment that includes a combination of different treatments provided in a specific sequence to treat the underlying cause of a condition. The process includes many elements developed specifically for the DMR Method, such as a progression of joint manipulation (Integrated Progressive Manipulation), a muscle massage and mobilization protocol (Dynamic Muscle Technique), and a progression of traction that were developed by the DMR Method clinical team. These elements work together synergistically to help patients achieve rapid and optimal results.

When should I come in for a DMR Method consult?

There are several ways of discerning whether you need a consult, including:

- Sciatica

- Chronic neck or back pain

- Upper or lower extremity pain, numbness, or weakness

- Headaches

- Herniated disc

- Stenosis

- Degenerative disc disease

- Spondylolisthesis

- Facet syndrome

- Whiplash

- If your back seems to be overly sensitive and gets aggravated or injured easily.

- If you've been recently injured.

- If spinal surgery has been recommended and it's not a medical emergency.

- If you've had spinal surgery and your symptoms have returned or worsened.

- If previous chiropractic, physical therapy, and other rehabilitation has failed to improve your condition.

Does the DMR Method treat conditions other than spinal conditions?

Yes. The DMR Method of evaluation and treatment is highly effective for non-spinal conditions. Because the DMR Method focuses on restoring mobility, alignment, and stability to joints and the supportive muscles and ligaments, non-spinal structural conditions such as sports injuries, rotator cuff syndrome, carpal tunnel syndrome, hip pain, and upper and lower extremity pain are treated with equal success.

Is the DMR Method covered by insurance, and can I use my health savings account to pay for treatment?

Yes. All of the clinical treatment components of the DMR Method are qualified for insurance coverage, but individual insurance benefits vary. We verify every patient's insurance benefits before we begin treatment and make sure they clearly understand what insurance will cover and what their personal financial responsibility will be. We will assist you in fulfilling any requirements your insurance or health savings account may have in order to maximize your benefits. Nutritional supplements, braces, supports, or other medical supplies are generally not covered by insurance.

Do I need a referral from my doctor for the DMR Method?

No, but depending on your health insurance policy guidelines, you may need a referral in order for parts of your treatment to be covered by insurance. We verify every patient's insurance coverage at the time of the initial consultation and help them acquire any necessary referrals to maximize their insurance benefits.

I've already tried chiropractic, physical therapy, and injections and none of it has worked. Why would this be any different?

The DMR Method is a unique combination of treatment modalities provided in a specific order by a team of physical therapists, chiropractors, and allied medical providers. Many patients may have already been treated with the individual components that comprise the DMR Method, but in the wrong order or the wrong combination.

Should I stop doing the exercises and stretches I was given by another healthcare provider?

Do only the self-care program given to you by your DMR Method provider in the order that they give it to you. Remember, the DMR Method is a treatment progression; performing parts of the treatment out of order can slow, plateau, or even block progress.

When I come in for treatment, how long are the appointments?

Regular visits are generally one hour; appointments that include an exam can last up to one-and-a-half hours. A typical visit will see you working with a tightly coordinated team of healthcare providers.

When I've completed the DMR Method, will I be completely better?

No. It takes eleven to eighteen months for ligaments and other supportive soft tissue to reach maximum strength. See "The Eleven-to-Eighteen-Month Rule" section in chapter 4 of this book. It's essential that you stay consistent with your self-care program and recommended clinical maintenance care during that time frame.

Do I really need to come in for treatment three times per week initially?

Yes. The DMR Method is a progression of care that focuses on the treatment of the underlying cause of a condition by improving mobility, alignment, and stability of the involved area. Maximal recovery requires consistency in both the frequency of corrective treatment and in the self-care program given to each patient. Think of the DMR Method as a training program for your spine; any fitness training program requires consistent repetition to achieve positive results. As your condition improves, treatment frequency will begin to taper off as you learn more advanced self-care.

When should I begin to see results from the DMR Method?

Depending upon your condition, you may feel some relief following the very first visit; or it could take a number of weeks to notice significant change.

Typically, symptoms tend to significantly improve within the first three weeks. Staying consistent with all the elements of the DMR Method will help ensure maximal results in the shortest period of time.

What if I have a vacation or other conflict that interrupts my treatment?

Communication is key. If your DMR Method providers are aware of an upcoming lapse of treatment, they will be able to tell you what you need to do to maintain your progress while you're away. If you are about to begin the DMR Method and have a conflict that will cause a lapse in treatment early on in your program, the providers may recommend that you wait until you are able to be consistent with clinical treatment before beginning your program. Consistency in the first three weeks of treatment is critical.

Can I still do the DMR Method if I've already had surgery?

Many patients who have successfully completed DMR Method treatment have previously had one or more surgeries. In general, these cases are more challenging and often require modifications to the normal treatment protocol. Sometimes we have to communicate with the surgeon who performed the surgery to get special direction or to learn more about the surgical procedure performed. When we accept a patient who has already had surgery, our goal is to provide safe treatment and prevent the need for more surgery.

I'm a doctor. One of my patients asked me if they should try the DMR Method. How can I learn more about it?

Visit DRMMethod.com, or read this book, especially chapters 4 and 6.

What if I get better faster than expected?

We progress every patient as rapidly as possible through the DMR Method treatment progression. That's why we have three treatment progressions: the Limited Protocol, the Progressed Protocol, and the Advanced Protocol (see chapter 4). When we initially evaluate patients, we do our best to recommend the right progression for their specific condition; if they progress more quickly or slowly, we modify their program to meet their unique needs. Regardless of the timing, every patient is directed through the three phases of recovery (relief, repair, and rehab) to optimize the three goals of treatment (mobility, alignment, and stability).

Do I need to keep coming in for any type of maintenance care after I complete the DMR Method?

The only form of maintenance care that's mandatory upon completion of the DMR Method is consistently following your self-care program, which includes stabilization exercises, stretches, proper body mechanics, and abiding by appropriate physical limitations. Some patients require periodic maintenance care that can include chiropractic treatment, traction, or physical therapy designed to support recovery. Appropriate maintenance care needs are identified by the patient, therapists, and doctors at the time of graduation from initial treatment.

If my leg hurts, why is my back the problem?

Sometimes the nerves extending from the lower part of the spine get irritated from a structural issue in the spine. Instead of experiencing low-back symptoms, the patient may experience symptoms in the area in which the irritated nerve is distributed. Treating the structural issue in the spine is essential to addressing the underlying cause of nerve irritation.

Is it okay for me to take pain medication or muscle relaxers while I'm doing the DMR Method?

In general, recovery is slowed and sometimes blocked by the use of medication to control symptoms. Masking symptoms with medication can make you prone to aggravation and re-injury because your body's ability to tell you when you're doing harmful physical activity is diminished. We recommend minimizing the use of medications; however, make sure to discuss this issue with any doctors who have provided you with prescriptions before making any change.

Can I use an inversion table or other home traction device to help my back?

When used properly, a home traction device can be of great benefit in your treatment or as a form of maintenance care following graduation from the DMR Method. However, in some cases, home traction is not recommended. Your DMR Method provider will tell you which form of home traction would be best for you and will also give you guidance on proper use.

I'm currently receiving the DMR Method but am not progressing as rapidly as other patients. How come?

Each patient's condition and speed of recovery are unique, so your progress may be slower than average. Many factors can influence the rate and extent of improvement, including:

- Inconsistency with self-care procedures, including appropriate physical limitations, using proper body mechanics, stretches, exercises, and supportive nutrition.
- Not being consistent with frequency of clinical care.
- Being overweight.
- Smoking.
- Excessive emotional stress.

You can work with your DMR Method providers to identify areas that need to be changed or modified in your treatment plan to maximize the speed and extent of improvement.

What if the DMR Method doesn't work?

We can't help everyone with the DMR Method, but for patients we accept for care, we are 96 percent successful in significantly decreasing symptoms and improving functional abilities. For those who are not candidates for the DMR Method, or who aren't responding to treatment, our goal is to make appropriate recommendations for other evaluation and treatment that will help them recover.

How can I participate in one of the DMR Method clinical case studies?

Many factors determine whether a patient is a candidate for one of the DMR Method clinical case studies. Your DMR Method provider will discuss this possibility with you and decide if you're a candidate for the current DMR Method case study.

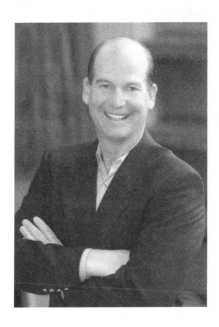

About Dr. Pete L'Allier

Dr. L'Allier completed his graduate studies at Northwestern Health Sciences University in 1990. After becoming a licensed and board-certified chiropractor the following year, Pete founded one of the first clinics in the country to offer chiropractors, physical therapists, occupational therapists, and medical doctors working together as an integrated team.

He is the founder and president of Hopkins Health & Wellness Center, he and his team created the DMR Method, a nonsurgical process of evaluation and treatment for neck and back pain. Dr. L'Allier is a healthcare researcher who has served as an associate clinical faculty member at Northwestern College of Chiropractic, has mentored numerous students and healthcare providers, and has been a speaker on topics of health and wellness for a number of corporations and organizations.

Dr. L'Allier is also the creator of School Survivor, a character-building and team-building program for children that has benefited thousands of elementary, middle school, and high school children. He and his wife, Jennifer, have two children and live on a hobby farm in Minnetrista, Minnesota.